EXPOSING

THE

SPIRITUAL ROOTS

OF

HIGH BLOOD PRESSURE

POWERFUL ANSWERS FOR
HEALING AND DISEASE PREVENTION

DR. HENRY W. WRIGHT

WHITAKER
HOUSE

Publisher's Note: This book is not intended to provide medical or psychological advice or to take the place of medical advice and treatment from your personal physician. Those who are having suicidal thoughts or who have been emotionally, physically, or sexually abused should seek help from a mental health professional or qualified counselor. Neither the publisher nor the author nor the author's ministry takes any responsibility for any possible consequences from any action taken by any person reading or following the information in this book. If readers are taking prescription medications, they should consult with their physicians and not take themselves off prescribed medicines without the proper supervision of a physician. Always consult your physician or other qualified health-care professional before undertaking any change in your physical regimen, whether fasting, diet, medications, or exercise.

All Scripture quotations are taken from the King James Version of the Holy Bible.

Boldface type in Scripture quotations indicates the author's emphasis. The forms LORD and GOD (in small capital letters) in Bible quotations represent the Hebrew name for God *Yahweh* (Jehovah), while *Lord* and *God* normally represent the name *Adonai*, in accordance with the Bible version used.

Exposing the Spiritual Roots of High Blood Pressure
Powerful Answers for Healing and Disease Prevention

Be in Health®, LLC
4178 Crest Highway, Thomaston, GA 30286
www.beinhealth.com
info@beinhealth.com

ISBN: 978-1-64123-752-9 • eBook ISBN: 978-1-64123-753-6
Printed in the United States of America
© 2021 by Be in Health®, LLC. All rights reserved.

Whitaker House
1030 Hunt Valley Circle • New Kensington, PA 15068
www.whitakerhouse.com

Library of Congress Control Number: 2021947930

1 2 3 4 5 6 7 8 9 10 11 **W** 28 27 26 25 24 23 22 21

CONTENTS

DISCLAIMER

We do not seek to be in conflict with any medical or psychiatric practice, or any church or its religious doctrines, beliefs, or practices. We are not part of medicine or psychology; we are working to make them more effective, believing that many human problems are fundamentally spiritual, with associated physiological and psychological manifestations. This information is intended for your general knowledge only, to give insight into disease, its problems, and possible solutions. It is not a substitute for medical advice or treatment from specific medical conditions or disorders. We do not diagnose or treat disease.

You should seek prompt medical care for any specific health issues. Treatment modalities around your specific health issues are between you and your physician. We are not responsible for a person's disease or their healing. We are administering the Scriptures and what they say about this subject, along with what the medical and scientific communities have observed in line with this insight. There is no guarantee any person will be healed or any disease prevented. The fruit of this teaching will come forth out of the application of the principles and the relationship between each person and God. Be in Health is patterned after 2 Corinthians 5:18–20, 1 Corinthians 12, Ephesians 4, and Mark 16:15–20.

FOREWORD

My husband, Dr. Henry W. Wright, was a brilliant man with a hunger for learning and an even stronger desire to serve God with all of his heart. He met the challenges of life with compassion, tough love, and his unique humor. It would be impossible to measure the impact he had on the lives of the people around him. His heart was to lead others to wholeness and peace in the love of God. He did his best to represent God's love in all that he did.

During his early years as a pastor, Henry's prayer was for answers to why physical healing from disease was not happening as often as it should in the church. That question, and God's answers, began his lifelong journey to exposing the spiritual roots of disease that were plaguing the body of Christ.

Henry spent decades researching biblical truths on what God said about healing, studying case histories of the people who came to the ministry for help, and learning about diseases and their effects on the human body from medical science. Together, we founded Be in Health and traveled throughout the United States and countries worldwide to teach biblical truths for overcoming diseases. The fantastic results were healing and restoration for tens of thousands of people across the globe. As the need for ministry increased, the For My Life Retreat was birthed. This impactful weeklong retreat on our church campus in Thomaston, Georgia, helps people understand the spiritual root causes of disease, apply the scriptural truths to their lives, and learn how to be set free!

Henry passed away in November 2019. Along with our family, church, and friends, I miss his presence every day. Shortly after Henry's passing, God spoke to my heart, "He's with Me, and he's good." Over five years ago, Henry and I, along with the Board of Elders, developed a plan to carry the biblical truths God had given him far into the future. Through Henry's relationship with the eldership and church body, we had a clear vision of how to move forward. Henry's vision was to establish generations of overcomers who would be restored—spirit, soul, and body—by God's Word and love.

Today, that is exactly what we are doing. The Be in Health team has expanded and continues to minister to thousands each month via our Thomaston, Georgia, campus, online seminars, mini-teachings, and conferences in cities across the country. The world is in great need of God's love and power to defeat the enemy and any diseases in their lives. I hope the biblical insights Henry deposited in this book help lead you in your journey of healing and restoration.

—*Donna Wright*

One

WHY AM I SICK?

Why am I sick?" "Why did this happen to me?" If you are fighting high blood pressure, you are searching everywhere for answers to these questions. At Be in Health, I have spent decades researching the *root cause of disease*. This is vital because people want answers to these questions: "Why am I sick?" "How can I be well?" Doesn't it make sense that we get down to the *root cause* that triggers disease in the first place? From there we can uproot it! Why? Because God's desire is for you to live in health and wholeness!

By God's grace, we have discovered answers to the root causes of disease that can put you on the road to healing and health. I want to state from the beginning that my research has revealed that approximately 80 percent of all chronic diseases have a *spiritual root cause*. Eighty percent is an astounding number! I believe that it is God's will to expose those spiritual roots and set you on the pathway to health. Because of what God has revealed in over 30 years of observing case studies, researching science, and studying His Word, thousands of people worldwide are free of their diseases and syndromes because they dealt with the root issues causing the manifestations. The healing answers that we will share in this book are from God's guidance and His Word and all the glory for these healings belongs to Him!

GOD'S PROMISES FOR HEALTH

God has given us many promises for health and healing. He meant for us to live in wholeness. "[I am the God] *who forgiveth all thine iniquities; who healeth all thy diseases*" (Psalm 103:3). "*Who his own self* [Jesus] *bare our sins in his own body on the tree, that we, being dead to sins, should live unto righteousness: by whose stripes ye were healed*" (1 Peter 2:24). Jesus also declared that healing was the "*children's bread.*" (See Matthew 15:26).

If God has promised us that our diseases can be healed, then why are we sick? Why are so many people, including Christians, still suffering with chronic illnesses—autoimmune diseases such as multiple sclerosis, rheumatoid arthritis, lupus, Graves' disease, diabetes 1, as well as cancer, diabetes 2, high blood pressure and heart disease, chronic depression, and so many more? To find the answers, we need to take a journey together to expose the spiritual roots of disease and discover how you can live in wholeness—spirit, soul, and body. My prayer is that this journey will fill you with peace and produce the understanding and wisdom that will bring you freedom from disease!

WHAT IS HIGH BLOOD PRESSURE?

Hypertension is the medical term for what is commonly called high blood pressure. Your blood pressure is determined by two variables: the amount of blood your heart pumps and the amount of resistance to blood flow in your arteries. The more blood your heart must pump, and the narrower your arteries, the higher your blood pressure. Blood pressure readings have two numbers. The top number, or systolic pressure, measures the pressure in your arteries when your heart beats. The bottom number, or diastolic pressure, measures the pressure in your arteries between the beats. Both numbers need to be in a healthy range for your heart to be protected from the damage of high blood pressure. A normal adult range is lower than 120 (top number) and lower than 80 (bottom number). As the numbers rise from there, you are diagnosed with high blood pressure. A reading of higher than 180 over 120 is considered a crisis stage which requires immediate medical attention.

Medical science has defined two types of high blood pressure. *Secondary* hypertension is diagnosed in individuals whose high blood pressure is caused by an underlying condition. Secondary hypertension tends to appear suddenly and often causes a higher blood pressure reading than primary hypertension. Various conditions can lead to secondary hypertension, including kidney disease, diabetes, sleep apnea, thyroid problems, and certain medications.

The other type of high blood pressure is referred to as *primary*, or essential, hypertension. Primary hypertension develops gradually over many years. For years, medical science has not listed a specific medical cause for this type of high blood pressure, although their recognition of the role of stress has increased in recent studies. In this book, our focus is on the spiritual roots of *primary hypertension*.

Your body produces a surge of hormones when you're in a stressful situation. These hormones increase your blood pressure by causing your heart to beat faster and your blood vessels to narrow. If this happens repeatedly, damage occurs. For primary hypertension, we have discovered that the spiritual roots are *fear, anxiety, and stress.*

As a result of these stress-related roots, the cell membrane (walls) of the arteries begin to stiffen and constrict causing a narrowing of the blood vessels near the heart. This results in a resistance to blood flow. As the blood backs up in the coronary blood vessels, it increases the pressure on the heart. The result is high blood pressure, which, if untreated, can lead to heart attack and stroke.

UNDERSTANDING THE ROOT CAUSE OF DISEASE

There is so much misunderstanding in the medical community and even in the church about the root cause of disease in mankind. In my research, I have studied what God has said in His Word very closely, and I have also spent years studying medical science. It's important to study the human body God has created as well as what He has declared in His Word about our bodies and health. Although some people have accused me of being against science, I'm indebted to it because it has enabled me to see things that I could not see otherwise.

Unfortunately, the blind side of science is that scientists and medical professionals tend to believe only what they can perceive with their five physical senses. The Bible gives us a much greater insight to see beyond what we can observe in the natural.

Answers to man's diseases and problems have been laid out in the Bible for over thirty-five hundred years. So why don't people read the Bible to discover those answers? That is what we are going to do in the following chapters. We will look at what God *and* science have to say about the root causes of and pathways to the recovery from disease—including high blood pressure. We will uncover the answers that you are searching for—to put you on the road to healing and health.

CAN GOD HEAL YOU?

I want to put your fears to rest that you cannot be cured of high blood pressure or other stress-related heart conditions. With God, all things are possible! (See, for example, Matthew 19:26.) There is complete healing and restoration possible for all diseases. By God's grace, at Be in Health, we have identified the spiritual roots of disease and successfully helped people overcome those root causes with amazing results of healing and recovery. They have found the pathway to true lasting healing that comes from God. According to Psalm 103, God heals all your diseases, redeems your life from the pit, crowns you with love, and makes you feel young all over again! That is the love of God! "*Who forgiveth all thine iniquities; who healeth all thy diseases; who redeemeth thy life from destruction; who crowneth thee with lovingkindness and tender mercies; who satisfieth thy mouth with good things; so that thy youth is renewed like the eagle's*" (Psalm 103:3–5).

Disease prevents you from having a full life; healing gets you back to normal and maybe even better than you were before your diagnosis. That is *A More Excellent Way*! You will learn from

God's Word how you can walk in healing and wholeness for the rest of your life!

CREATED IN HIS IMAGE

The Bible tells us in Genesis that God created man in His own image. *"And God said, Let us make man in our image, after our likeness…So God created man in his own image, in the image of God created he him; male and female created he them"* (Genesis 1:26–27). If we live as God designed us, we will be changed back into His image and thrive. We will function at our highest level. However, if we follow paths or ways of thinking about ourselves that are not in agreement with His plan, we lose our identity in God and may open a door to disease in our bodies. God is the author of what He has created: you. God is the sustainer of what He has created: you. So, if we dismiss God as part of the equation in our healing, what have we got? We have cut ourselves off from the source of our answer to the recovery and healing of disease.

God's desire as our heavenly Father is to form us back into our true identity as His children, in His image, and according to His nature. To understand who we are, we need to know who God is. First and foremost, He is our Father. Jesus was sent to the earth to restore our relationship with our heavenly Father. *"For if, when we were enemies, we were **reconciled to God by the death of his Son**, much more, being reconciled, we shall be saved by his life"* (Romans 5:10). First John tells us that *"God is love"* (1 John 4:8, 16). And we reflect God's nature within us when we manifest the fruit of the Holy Spirit in our lives. *"The fruit of the Spirit is*

WHY AM I SICK? 15

love, joy, peace, longsuffering, gentleness, goodness, faith, meekness, temperance" (Galatians 5:22–23)—all attributes of a loving God.

Psalm 139:14–15 tells us that God the Father thoughtfully and carefully designed and created each one of us. *"I will praise thee; for I am fearfully and wonderfully made: marvellous are thy works; and that my soul knoweth right well. My substance was not hid from thee, when I was made in secret, and curiously wrought in the lowest parts of the earth."* We are each designed with a specific personality, unique characteristics, and our own purpose and place that are prepared for us in His family if we will accept it. We were not created or called to be anyone other than ourselves. Each person needs to settle in their own heart that they are fearfully and wonderfully made in the image of God, not in anyone else's image. God does not make accidents.

KEEP TRACKING WITH US STEP-BY-STEP

In *Exposing the Spiritual Roots of High Blood Pressure*, you will recognize the areas in life that can separate you from your identity as a child of God. The Father wants to help us realign our hearts with His heart. We must learn to accept what He says about us as truth. In this journey, we will answer many questions along the way. How can this loss of your identity in God the Father lead to disease? How did the spiritual roots of disease begin? What are the specific spiritual roots of high blood pressure, and how have they invaded your life?

In the early chapters, we will expose the unseen forces that trigger all disease from within and how you can overcome them. You will recognize the battleground that paves the way for disease, and how to apply the Word of God to receive your healing. In the later chapters, we will expose the specific spiritual root causes of high blood pressure, highlighting the case studies of people who have experienced healing from their disease. Your healing is what this journey is all about.

Since there is a great deal to learn about the spiritual roots of disease, I will take you step-by-step to truly understand how you can walk in healing and wholeness for the rest of your life! Please don't try to get ahead of yourself. Read the truths in this book one step at a time. The Bible encourages us to learn by establishing a *firm foundation* and then building upon it *one precept* (guiding principle) or line at a time. *"For precept must be upon precept, precept upon precept; line upon line, line upon line; here a little, and there a little"* (Isaiah 28:9–10). Keep tracking with us closely throughout this journey—your freedom from disease may depend on it!

Two

WHAT IS THE SPIRITUAL ROOT OF DISEASE?

Did you know that you are a creative miracle of God? We have already recognized that human beings were created in God's image. God is a triune Being—Three in One—Father, Son, and Holy Spirit. In God's divine plan, He created us with three essential parts as well—*spirit, soul,* and *body.* The Bible states clearly, *"And the very God of peace sanctify you **wholly;** and I pray God your whole **spirit** and **soul** and **body** be preserved blameless unto the coming of our Lord Jesus Christ"* (1 Thessalonians 5:23).

*"May the God of peace sanctify you **wholly.**"* That word here is not H-O-L-Y. Even though the word *sanctified* does mean HOLY, the King James version of this verse says sanctified *"wholly."* W-H-O-L-L-Y. Completely, every part of us—*spirit, soul, and body*—sanctified and whole for His glory. You are a spirit, you have a soul, and you live in a body; you are a triune being. We need to understand this vital truth so that we can be healed and whole. How does this work?

First, we have a body. Our body is like our house—we live inside of it. Some of us have fancy roofs, some of us have thatched roofs, some have no roofs at all. We like to focus on the outward part—the body. You know there's nothing wrong with making our houses look nice. After all, we paint our homes, put shutters on them, plant flowers around them, and enjoy the beauty. We do the same thing with our bodies—we live in our bodies, and we often dress them up. The way our bodies feel impacts us power-fully. We focus on our bodies because that is what we experience with our five senses. So, the body is what we see, but it is only one part of our being.

Second, we have a soul. God created men and women with a soul. Our soul is comprised of our mind, will, and emotions. The way we view and experience the world with our minds and emotions is an integral part of who we are and has a significant effect on our bodies. We are greatly impacted at the soul level. Science has recognized this for a number of years with some-thing called the mind-body connection. "The mind-body con-nection is the link between a person's thoughts, attitudes, and behaviors and their physical health. While scientists have long understood that our emotions can affect our bodies, we're just now beginning to understand how emotions influence health and longevity."[1] "Mounting evidence for the role of the mind in dis-ease and healing is leading to a greater acceptance of mind-body medicine."[2] However, science doesn't recognize the third part of

---

1. Lakshmi Menezes, MD, "What Is the Mind-Body Connection?" Florida Medical Clinic blog, August 24, 2020, https://www.floridamedicalclinic.com/blog/what-is-the-mind-body-connection/.
2. Vicki Brower, "Mind-Body Research Moves Towards the Mainstream," EMBO reports, v. 7(4), April 2006, https://www.ncbi.nlm.nih.gov/pmc/articles/PMC1456909/.

our being—our spirit—and that acceptance of the spirit-soul-body relationship is key in the understanding of and fight against disease.

Third, we have a spirit. The most important part of our creation as humans is our *spirit*. This is the part of our human makeup that science doesn't recognize, and sometimes the church doesn't recognize it, either. The medical community focuses on our body, and they understand that we have a soul, but the spirit is ignored completely. Why is it important that we recognize the existence of this third part of our being? Because so many chronic diseases have their root cause or beginning in our spirits!

The biblical truth is that the *real* you is not your physical body, no matter how much you fix it up! Your body is just what you see with your five physical senses. There is so much more to you! God's Word reveals that the greatest impact on who we are is from within, at the *spirit* level. Our *whole* man—spirit, soul, and body—must be well to live in health. Now, I see three different perspectives on the root causes of disease: those of the medical community, of many in the church, and of the Word of God. We will look at these three different perspectives a little more closely.

WHAT DOES THE MEDICAL COMMUNITY SAY?

What does the medical community say about the root cause of disease? The truth is that doctors are at a loss for how and why many diseases begin. In medical textbooks, a large number of diseases are listed with the name of the disease, the body parts affected, the diagnosis, the prognosis, and the protocols. At the end of these journal entries, a specific medical phrase is inserted:

"etiology unknown." *Etiology* comes from the Greek and means "root cause" or "giving a reason for." The medical community knows they can see the disease, they can diagnose it, and they can track it, but they don't know or understand what triggers it.

All autoimmune diseases are catalogued as having an unknown etiology. That would include the more than 80 auto-immune diseases, including the most well-known ones: multiple sclerosis, rheumatoid arthritis, lupus, Graves' disease, Crohn's disease, and psoriasis. This is true for other non-autoimmune diseases, as well, such as chronic fatigue syndrome, fibromyalgia, and irritable bowel syndrome. With any disease that is considered incurable, the best the medical community can do is offer "disease management"—a combination of pills, therapies, or surgeries to keep the disease under control and hopefully extend the patient's life.

Please believe me—I am not against doctors or science! I have spent decades studying what medical science knows about the intricate human body that God has created. I am very thankful for what I have learned. But I do not want to just offer you "disease management"! By God's help, I want to expose the spiritual roots of disease and offer true health—spirit, soul, and body! That's because the God I serve—He represents your wholeness!

WHAT DOES THE CHURCH SAY?

Unfortunately, many Christians are often confused about healing and health. They know that the Bible gives us promises for healing, such as Psalm 103:2–3: "*Bless the* Lord…*who forgiveth all thine iniquities; who healeth all thy diseases.*" But then they ask a very fair question, "Why aren't we seeing more people being healed?"

Christian leaders don't know the answer to this question, and so doctrines are created that contradict the Bible, such as the argument that "supernatural healing ended with the first apostles." Discouragement, doubt, and unbelief creep into the church. Without answers to the question of healing, some Christians simply resign themselves to illness. They even begin to ask, "Is God the one who brings disease? Is God just testing us or purifying us?" But that's not what the Word of God says! The Bible says that what God desires for us is *health and wholeness.*

The apostle John wrote, *"Beloved, I wish **above all things** that thou mayest prosper and be in health, even as thy soul prospereth"* (3 John 2). Now, I ask you, is there anything more "all" than *"all"*? John says he wishes for health above *all* things. Jesus Himself stated, *"I am come that they might have life, and that they might have it more abundantly"* (John 10:10). Abundant life includes freedom from disease. I want to be very clear here. I believe God's perfect will is not just to heal you. His perfect will is that you *don't get sick in the first place!* But if you are sick, then His healing is yours!

I ask people who are confused about God and health, "Why would God bring disease? Why would God destroy what He created?" God is not trying to destroy you! After He created Adam and Eve, He looked at them and proclaimed, "It is very good." (See Genesis 27–31.) He never said, "Look at those diseased beings that I just created!" No, God does not give us disease. In Hosea 4: 6, the Lord warns, *"My people are destroyed for lack of knowledge."* This verb in the Hebrew is written in the present tense, so it still applies to us today: *"My people **are** [**being**] destroyed for lack of knowledge."* God's people are suffering *in the present* because they don't have the knowledge that they need in order to be in health!

In the church, we need *wholeness* centers—places where we can be healed in our *spirit, soul, and body.* We shouldn't just farm our people out to a medical world that doesn't understand God and doesn't understand how He desires to heal us and make us whole. If we want this wholeness, we must recognize the truth of how God created us.

WHAT DOES GOD'S WORD SAY?

The Bible is clear! God wants to bring truth and freedom to us in our spirits, our souls, and our bodies. Again, *"I pray God your whole **spirit and soul and body** be preserved blameless unto the coming of our Lord Jesus Christ"* (1 Thessalonians 5:23).

In a world that questions whether truth even exists and often redefines truth as relative to personal whims, God's truth remains the same. It is His Word—the Bible. The Bible states that *all* of the Scriptures are God-inspired: *"All scripture is given by inspiration of God, and is profitable for doctrine, for reproof, for correction, for instruction in righteousness"* (2 Timothy 3:16). Since the Bible contains God's truth, then that is where we will find our answers for health and wholeness. That is where we will find the root cause of disease and how we may be restored to health.

Since the healing promises are given over and over again by God in His Word, why are so many sons and daughters of the

Father suffering with as much disease as the rest of the world? Have God's promises changed? Never. The promises of God give us the foundation and the faith to stand against disease. If you take the promises out of the Bible, what do you have? Nothing for your faith to believe with or stand on. Your faith comes directly from hearing God's infallible Word. *"So then faith cometh by hearing, and hearing by the word of God"* (Romans 10:17). You hear His Word, and faith rises within your spirit, and you embrace that faith. Faith is for today; faith is for right now. Healing and health are for right now.

Then what is the disconnect? If God's Word says that healing is the children's bread (see Matthew 15:22–29), that Jesus paid for the curse of sin on the cross (see Galatians 3:13), and that by His stripes, or wounds, we are healed (see Isaiah 53:5), then what has happened to us? Where have things gone wrong?

SEPARATION IS THE SPIRITUAL ROOT OF DISEASE

As I said earlier, after more than thirty years of research and experience with thousands of individuals, I am convinced that the root cause of about 80 percent of all chronic disease is spiritual. And that spiritual root is the direct result of separation in our lives on three very important levels:

1. Separation from God, His Word, His person, and His love

2. Separation from yourself by not accepting yourself and struggling with self-hatred, guilt, and shame

3. Separation from others by a breach of relationships

In the Bible, the First and Second Great Commandments are the foundation for this truth. When Jesus was asked which of the commandments was the greatest, He answered, *"Thou shalt love the Lord thy God with all thy heart, and with all thy soul, and with all thy mind. This is the first and great commandment. And the second is like unto it, Thou shalt love thy neighbour as thyself. On these two commandments hang all the law and the prophets"* (Matthew 22:37–40). With these two great commandments, God reveals the importance of love and acceptance without separation. First, love God Almighty with all of your being; second, love yourself because God created you in His love; third, love your neighbor with the same love as you love yourself because God created your neighbor, as well. When we don't obey these commandments to love, our disobedience brings on a critical separation that leads to the spiritual roots of disease and misery in our lives.

SEPARATION FROM OUR HEAVENLY FATHER

The first root of disease is separation from God. Mankind—that includes Christians—is diseased most of all because we are *separated from God, His Word, and His love.* We must realign ourselves with the Father, embracing the truth of His love for us. Jesus showed us the deep love of the Father by dying on the cross for our eternal redemption. *"For God so loved the world, that he gave his only begotten Son…"* (John 3:16). The Bible assures us of God's love: *"And we have known and believed **the love that God hath to us**. God is love; and he that dwelleth in love dwelleth in God and God in him"* (1 John 4:16). To be free and healed, you must believe God's Word that He truly *loves you.*

Unfortunately, "religion" has made God the Father seem unapproachable. It is easier to focus our love on Jesus as our Savior because He showed His love for us on the cross. People may feel more connected to Jesus. But Jesus came to this earth specifically to reconcile us to our Father—to take our sin upon Himself so that we would not be separated from the Father again. *"Now all these things are of God, who hath reconciled us to himself by Jesus Christ, and hath given to us the ministry of reconciliation"* (2 Corinthians 5:18).

It is the Father's heart for you to know how precious you are to Him. He refers to you as His beloved. *"Put on therefore, as the elect of God, holy and beloved…"* (Colossians 3:12). *"I will call them my people, which were not my people; and her beloved, which was not beloved"* (Romans 9:25). When Philip asked Jesus, *"Show us the Father"* (John 14:8), Jesus replied, *"He that hath seen me hath seen the Father"* (John 14:9). How Jesus taught, spoke, and acted was a reflection of the Father. That means it was the Father's love for us that Jesus healed the multitudes, rebuked evil spirits, fed the thousands, raised loved ones from the dead.

Sometimes we have a disconnect with God's love because our earthly father was not a good representation of the heavenly Father. Many of us stumble over the love of the Father because we never heard our earthly father say that he loved us. All around the world, people in our conferences have admitted that they never heard their father say those three simple words: "I love you." That was my personal experience as well. As a result, we have a problem understanding our identity as sons or daughters of our heavenly Father. We become fractured in our true identity.

This is a disease maker. You don't want to be separated from your heavenly Father for any reason.

One of the things I've done for years to help people deal with the damage done by an earthly father is to go through something I call The Father's Love Ministry. If you never hear your earthly father say, "I love you," I'm asking you to just open your heart and receive these words for your life:

> On behalf of the father that did not, could not, or would not—or maybe just didn't know how to—tell you that he loves you; on behalf of that father, I want to take responsibility for your life. On behalf of that father, will you forgive him for not telling you, "I love you"? I am so sorry for his silence and the junk and the hardness that may have injured you and left you feeling stranded on the inside when you needed him so much.

> Now, on behalf of that father, I want to tell you these words for your life: "I love you. I am so proud of you. I am glad that you were born. And you are a good son; you are a good daughter."

Embrace these words with all your heart.

SEPARATION FROM OURSELVES AND OTHERS

"And the second [great commandment] *is like unto it, Thou shalt love thy neighbour as thyself"* (Matthew 22:39).

The second root of disease is separation from ourselves. I discovered that it is impossible to love yourself if you have not accepted the Father's love for you. I have seen thousands of people over the last three-plus decades battle intensely with self-hatred, self-loathing, self-bitterness, and guilt. Not accepting the Father's love and hating yourself instead is a deep-rooted lie from the enemy that carries with it many grievous diseases and disorders. If this is your struggle, you must learn to accept yourself in your relationship with God and love yourself as God sees you, not embracing the deception of self-hatred and guilt. God loves you! He declares it in His Word, as we have already seen. This will be a vital link on this journey to identify the spiritual root of disease.

The third root of disease is separation from others. This flings the door wide-open to spiritually rooted disease. Unforgiveness and bitterness can become a root deep inside you that defiles those around you and makes your body extremely susceptible to disease. The Bible warns us, "[Look] *diligently lest any man fail of the grace of God; lest **any root of bitterness** spring up to trouble you, and thereby many be defiled"* (Hebrews 12:15).

Bitterness is a deeply rooted sin because you consider yourself to be God in the situation, judging right from wrong and choosing not to forgive. It is an ugly sin that corrodes like acid, eating away at your soul. First it poisons the mind and then the body. Be kind to yourself. Make peace with your family members, church leaders, brothers and sisters in Christ, and anyone else who has injured or offended you. God commands it, and He knows that it will destroy your life if you live in unforgiveness and bitterness.

Now, if the root of 80 percent of chronic disease is spiritual, then 80 percent of all healing starts with *the restoration of our relationships with God, ourselves, and others!* How do I know this? Decades of the intense study of disease and thousands of case studies later, I have seen the successful result of applying the truths you are about to learn. We will unfold this restoration of our relationships to God, ourselves, and others in great detail as we continue on our journey to healing.

HEALED FROM DISEASE

Right now, I'd like to share the case history of a woman named Christine who came to us at Be in Health to find answers for her healing of Graves' disease.

> Over sixteen years ago, I was diagnosed with Graves' disease, an autoimmune disease where your body attacks the tissue in your healthy thyroid as though it were an enemy disease. The result is an overactive thyroid producing too much of the hormone thyroxine. I struggled for fourteen years with Graves' disease, and I had five miscarriages because of it. During my "thyroid storms," when I was overcome with irregular heartbeats, tremors, anxiety, and confusion, I felt like I was losing my mind. My older children thought I was going crazy, too! I was so weak—no strength at all. At that point, it seemed like my life was coming to an end even though I was only in my early forties. I felt hopeless.

> During the years I struggled with Graves' disease, I tried many avenues to be healed. When the doctors and endocrinologists couldn't find a cure, I turned to

alternative methods, including essential oils, naturo-path doctors, and fifteen supplements that I would take every day. The results were the same. I was incurable.

Thankfully, I had a friend who had been to a For My Life retreat. One day, she told me, "I think you have a spirit of fear." I didn't know what she was talking about, but I was curious. I traveled from Colorado to the Be in Health center in Georgia. I didn't expect to be cured; I just thought they might be able to make me feel a little better. But I was wrong. God had so much more for me there. The whole restoration process of bringing me back to the Father's love was intense. I struggled to believe that I was God's beloved. I kept confessing it to my family so that I could hear my own words. Once I finally believed it for myself, that's when my healing began to come forth speedily.

I left the For My Life retreat in March. In May of that year, I had an appointment with my naturopath doctor in Arizona who had been running all of my blood tests. The doctor was astonished at my test results. She walked back into the examination room and said, "Christine, I don't know what you've done, but your thyroid is totally normal! Your TSH (thyroid-stimulating hormone), T3, and T4 hormone levels are all normal!" The doctor ordered a new ultrasound, and my goiter had disappeared completely! I had spent thousands of dollars traveling to clinics, experimenting with natural remedies, and taking those fifteen daily supplements over the years. My healing came with no medications, no supplements! My greatest blessing? I had a baby at the age of forty-six! He's the perfect addition to our family!

I have seen true restoration in my life. God didn't just hand me back the years I lost; He greatly restored those years to me. I feel full of life. I feel younger than I have for years and have so much more energy than I ever did—and an abiding peace and joy. The main thing, truly the overriding message, has been the restoration with my heavenly Father. I really know that I am His beloved.

—Christine

Three

WHERE DISEASE BEGAN

In all three of the spiritual separations that we just read about, we are tempted by an unseen enemy to reject our love for God, ourselves, and others. This unseen enemy who finds a place to sneak in to destroy us is Satan, whom Jesus called *"the thief... [who comes] to kill, to steal, and to destroy"* (John 10:10). The apostle Paul warns us not to be *"ignorant of* [Satan's] *devices"* (2 Corinthians 2:11). The word *"devices"* refers to the devil's methods, mythologies, and practices—the way he has been scheming to destroy God's people since the garden of Eden. When you embrace the enemy's lies, you end up suffering at his hands. You need to know how the enemy is doing it. You need to understand his devices so that you can cut him off at the pass in your life! We need to look at how this happens and how disease began in the first place.

Do you know how many diseases there are? Over three thousand diseases and disorders have been identified to date! Where did they come from? They didn't come from God. When He created man, He created something that was very good, but then something came along to interfere—something that wasn't good. This is the enemy lurking around, whose sole ambition is to interfere with God's plan and destroy the people God has created. His name is Satan, and the goal of his dark kingdom is to steal, kill, and destroy God's people on earth.

HOW DISEASE ENTERED THE WORLD

Let's start at the beginning—with Adam and Eve.

According to Genesis, chapter two, Adam walked in the cool of the evening with his Creator before Eve came on the scene. Just before Eve was created, Adam was given the first law from God. *"And the LORD God commanded the man, saying, Of every tree of the garden thou mayest freely eat: but of the tree of the knowledge of good and evil, thou shalt not eat of it: for in the day that thou eatest thereof thou shalt surely die"* (Genesis 2:16–17).

In the garden of Eden, Satan, the great deceiver, came to Eve and changed the Word of God. *"Now the serpent was more subtil [deceitful] than any beast of the field which the LORD God had made. And he said unto the woman, Yea, hath God said, Ye shall not eat of every tree of the garden?"* (Genesis 3:1). In other words, "Is this what God really said?" When Eve replied that God said they would die if they ate the fruit of one specific tree, Satan lied to contradict God's Word. *"And the serpent said unto the woman, Ye shall not surely die: for God doth know that in the day ye eat thereof, then your eyes shall be opened, and ye shall be as gods, knowing good and evil"* (Genesis 3:4–5). In other words, he whispered the great deception we still hear today: "God lied to you…there's really a better plan."

You know what happened next. Eve broke off the fruit, ate it, and then handed it to her husband who was standing right beside her. She repeated the enemy's lie— "Adam, we won't die; our eyes will be open to good and evil. It's going to make us wise!"—and he ate. Immediately, their spiritual eyes were opened; but at that moment, wisdom didn't flood them—evil did. They saw their nakedness before a holy God, and they hid from Him in fear. Adam, son of God, was suddenly afraid of the One whom he had walked with in perfect fellowship.

As evening approached, it was time for the Lord to meet with them. Genesis chapter three tells us that the Lord came looking, calling out something like this: "Where are you, Adam?" Adam finally had enough nerve to answer, "Here we are, Lord! Out here in the bushes." "Why are you hiding from Me, Adam?" "Because, Lord, we are naked." Now, read the words of the Lord in Genesis 3:11: *"And he [God] said, Who told thee that thou wast naked?"* God knew why they were hiding. He knew it was Satan who had seduced Adam and Eve and was now overwhelming them with thoughts of fear, guilt, and shame. But He wanted to know if Adam knew who had come to destroy him and his perfect communion with God.

This was the beginning of Adam and Eve's journey into a life of temptation and sin. When Adam and Eve rebelled and disobeyed the first law of God, sin and death—both spiritual and physical—entered the world. Death and disease came to this planet because of their disobedience. As a result, sin, disease, and death have passed from generation to generation, and we are still battling them to this day. This is the origin of disease.

Thank God that He had a plan to save us from what Satan meant for our total destruction. He had a plan through His Son Jesus to redeem a people who would love Him. God gave us a plan for our eternal salvation through the death and resurrection of Jesus Christ. He also gave us a plan to defeat Satan's schemes in our lives on earth. So why aren't Christians always following the plan?

THERE ARE TWO KINGDOMS

This account of Adam and Eve reveals a vital biblical truth: disease is no happenstance; it is a planned event by our spiritual enemy, Satan, and his dark kingdom. Many Christians have forgotten that we have a hidden enemy who is after our destruction. Remember the Scripture verse that says, *"My people are destroyed for lack of knowledge"* (Hosea 4:6)? God wasn't speaking just to the Old Testament saints here. I see this same lack of knowledge in the modern church today. People are ignorant of spiritual warfare.

The spirit world is a place where intelligent beings exist that do not have bodies in a physical sense. There are two kingdoms in this invisible world. There is the kingdom of God, which the Father rules from heaven. Heaven is not far away; it's just on the other side of what we can see, in a different dimension. Then there's the kingdom of darkness, which is inhabited by fallen spiritual beings and ruled by the ex-Archangel, Satan. That kingdom may not seem real in our "modern age," but it is clearly defined in the Bible for our benefit.

Jesus spoke with a great awareness of this evil kingdom when He said, *"And if Satan cast out Satan, he is divided against himself; how shall then his kingdom stand?"* (Matthew 12:26). Jesus accused the Pharisees of siding with evil: *"Ye are of your father the devil, and the lusts of your father ye will do. He was a murderer from the beginning, and abode not in the truth, because there is no truth in him. When he speaketh a lie, he speaketh of his own: for he is a liar, and the father of it"* (John 8:44).

The apostle Paul also warned us that our battle in life is not against flesh and blood that we can see. *"For we wrestle not against flesh and blood, but against principalities, against powers, against the rulers of the darkness of this world, against spiritual wickedness in high places"* (Ephesians 6:12). Your war is not with others. Your war is not even with yourself. Your war is with an evil kingdom filled with principalities, powers, spiritual wickedness in high places, and the rulers of the darkness of this world that you cannot see with your physical eyes.

Just like Adam and Eve, your war is with a hidden enemy who wants to form you into his image, but that image is the image of disease and death. Adam and Eve embraced that image. Jesus Christ's image is the image of wholeness and life. You must learn to embrace Jesus and His image! It is vital to our lives and our health that we understand the biblical truth that two kingdoms exist in the spiritual world: one of darkness and one of light. Jesus sent Paul to the people *"to open their eyes, and to turn them from darkness to light, and from the power of Satan unto God"* (Acts 26:18). There is great warfare between these two kingdoms. When we don't understand what is going on in the spirit world, we become victims of our own ignorance.

YOU ARE NOT YOUR DISEASE!

Don't embrace the spirit of death. God has created you with a purpose and a plan. God has created you to live. It is the enemy who wants to overthrow the plan that God has created for you. *You are not your disease.* Remind yourself: "I may *have* a disease, but I *am not* a disease!" Don't call it "my disease." There is sin that has been tormenting you, but you are not the sin. You are a child of God! Accept the Father's great love for you; He has called you to be His own! *"Yea, I have loved thee with an everlasting love: therefore with lovingkindness have I drawn thee"* (Jeremiah 31:3). You are not the problem; the devil is. Stop listening to him!

My desire is to open your eyes to God's truth concerning the spiritual root of all disease and the freedom from disease that can be yours. I want you to join me in this walk of freedom. I want you to embrace life! I want you to defeat everything that God hates. I don't want to offer you a counterfeit of humanism. I want to offer you the truth from God's Word. *"Ye shall know the truth, and the truth shall make you free"* (John 8:32). I want you to live in freedom from the bondage and the curse of disease. Satan may have evil devices, but God shows us how we can defeat him and be in health.

HOW DO WE CHOOSE LIFE?

"I have set before you life and death, blessing and cursing: therefore choose life" (Deuteronomy 30:19). Moses presented this decision to God's people thousands of years ago, and we must make this same decision today—the choice between life and death,

blessings and curses. During his final address to the Israelites, Moses shared this powerful message from God. *"I call heaven and earth to record this day against you, that I have set before you **life and death, blessing and cursing***: *therefore choose life, that both thou and thy seed may live"* (Deuteronomy 30:19).

Life and blessings come from obedience to God. *"And it shall come to pass, **if thou shalt hearken diligently** unto the voice of the* LORD *thy God, to observe and to do all his commandments which I command thee this day, that the* LORD *thy God will set thee on high above all nations of the earth. And **all these blessings** shall come on thee, and overtake thee, if thou shalt hearken unto the voice of the* LORD *thy God"* (Deuteronomy 28:1). Look what God was promising! If they chose God's voice—*if they chose life*—they would be *"high above all nations of the earth,"* and they would be *"overtaken"* by more blessings than they could count. These blessings would overtake them *if* they listened to and obeyed the Lord. What a promise!

However, that was not the end of Moses's message. He followed it with a warning that the Israelites should never forget. *"But it shall come to pass, **if thou wilt not hearken** unto the voice of the* LORD *thy God, to observe to do all his commandments and his statutes which I command thee this day; that **all these curses** shall come upon thee and overtake thee"* (Deuteronomy 28:15). For the next forty-three verses, Moses described the curses—the disastrous events and diseases—that would overtake God's chosen people if they chose not to listen to Him and not to follow His commandments. By their disobedience, they would open themselves to the enemy's lies, which would lead to curses…and many of those curses are diseases.

Please understand me—I am not into legalism. I am into something called heart change. I'm into understanding the Word of God because it is truth—truth that brings us freedom from disease. Some people say that the Old Testament is not for Christians today. However, in the Old Testament, God says that He will bless *"them that love me and keep my commandments"* (Deuteronomy 5:10). In the New Testament, Jesus said to His disciples, *"If ye love me, keep my commandments"* (John 14:15.) The apostle John wrote, *"For this is the love of God, that we keep his commandments: and his commandments are not grievous"* (1 John 5:3). Throughout the Bible, God asks us to obey His commandments because it is His will, and also because those commandments have been created for our good, our protection, and our health.

WHAT EXACTLY IS A CURSE?

Disobeying God can bring a curse of disease. What exactly is a curse? People are afraid of the word, and it isn't something we talk about much in the church today. I decided to do a little word study of the Hebrew word for *curse* based on Deuteronomy 28. The first word I found for the meaning of curse was *vilification*. Vilification starts with the same letters as the word *villain*. The minute I saw the word *villain*, I thought of Jesus's words about Satan. Jesus said, *"The thief cometh not, but for to steal, and to kill, and to destroy: I am come that they might have life, and that they might have it more abundantly"* (John 10:10). That thief—Satan— is the enemy, the villain in our lives. My study also revealed that a curse is *an abatement* of the blessing. The word *abatement* means "lessening" or "reduction." So, the villain, who is Satan, comes to abate or reduce the strength of our blessings from God. The curse is the work of this villain.

In Moses's address to the Israelites in Deuteronomy, chapter twenty-eight, we can find every class of disease known to man. God called these diseases the result of a curse—an abatement of His blessing. In my ministry, I began to encounter far too many New Testament believers who were plagued with the exact same diseases as those listed in Deuteronomy. They had autoimmune disease, they had heart disease, they had digestive disorders, they had cancer, they had depression. I began to wonder, "Why are these biological and psychological disorders called a curse in the Old Testament, but the same things that are found in New Testament covenant saints aren't called a curse?"

CAN CURSES AFFECT CHRISTIANS TODAY?

I am very serious about this. Our world, and even the church, is filled with every work of the devil found in Deuteronomy 28 which is called the curse. Disease, syndromes, depression, anxiety disorders, family discord, job loss—it's all there. Our lives are under attack, not just our bodies. That brings up an important question: Can curses affect Christians today? The Bible tells us that a curse without cause—without a reason for being there—cannot affect us. *"As the bird by wandering, as a swallow by flying, so a curse without cause shall not alight"* (Proverbs 20:2).

Didn't Christ end the curse from Adam and Eve by His death on the cross? *"Christ hath redeemed us from the curse of the law, being made a curse for us"* (Galatians 3:13). Yes, He did, and He made it possible for us to live in righteousness and wholeness by His death and resurrection. Then how can Christians, who are covered by the blood of the Lamb, be under the burden of a curse? It is because the effects of a curse are *a result of disobedience to God's Word*, and Christians can be just as disobedient to God's Word as the Old Testament believers were. Curses can alight because we give them the permission to do it!

Now, I am not talking about Christians being possessed by an evil spirit. I am not talking about losing your salvation. I am talking about servitude to the enemy. It means that you are serving the law of sin presented to you by Satan rather than serving the law of God. A curse that has no cause cannot affect a Christian's salvation. But it can wreak havoc in our lives if we give the villain who is behind that curse permission. Satan doesn't have all power. He can only touch you with your permission when you embrace the law of sin. How can we give the devil this permission? *By disobeying God and His Word and obeying the law of sin instead.* But God has provided the pathway to our freedom from the law of sin.

God's thinking is superior, and Satan's thinking is inferior. "*Ye are of God little children and have overcome them; because greater is he that is in you, than he that is in the world*" (1 John 4:4). Greater is God who is in you than the enemy who is in the world. You choose whom you will serve. God will not leave you or forsake you as you take this journey to freedom! Keep on tracking with me on this road to your health and wholeness. "*Be strong and be of good courage; fear not, nor be afraid of them: for the LORD thy God, he it is that doth go with thee; he will not fail thee, nor forsake thee!*" (Deuteronomy 31:6). Don't be afraid of this battle. God is our victory!

Four

WINNING THE WAR WITHIN

Did you know that as Christians we can still have a war raging within? Paul, an apostle of Jesus Christ, confessed that there was a war within him—two laws battling for his soul—the law of God and the law of sin. Paul declared:

> For the good that I would I do not: but the evil which I would not, that I do. Now if I do that I would not, it is no more I that do it, but sin that dwelleth in me. I find then a law, that, when I would do good, evil is present with me. For I delight **in the law of God** after the inward man: but I **see another law in my members**, warring against the law of my mind, and bringing me into **captivity to the law of sin** which is in my members. O wretched man that I am! who shall deliver me from the body of this death? **I thank God through Jesus Christ our Lord.**   (Romans 7:19–25)

PAUL'S WAR WITHIN

The battle between the law of sin and the law of God that happened in Paul two thousand years ago is still happening in us today. You may ask, "I thought we weren't under the law anymore?" When Paul talks about the law of God here, he isn't speaking about rules; he is referring to God's nature. It is a reflection of God's righteousness. God is good; God is love; God is justice; God is mercy; God is forgiveness; God is faithfulness. These things and more are His nature and His righteousness—the law that God promised to write on our hearts. *"I will put my laws into their mind, and write them in their hearts: and I will be to them a God, and they shall be to me a people"* (Hebrews 8:10).

On the other side of the war is the law of sin, which is the nature of Satan: rebellion, lawlessness, hatred, murder, evil, and falsehoods. The law of sin will always attempt to compete with the law of God through temptation. In this battle, Paul is saying, "The things that I wish I wouldn't do, that's what I do; and the good that I want to do, I don't do it." Well, that sounds just like us, doesn't it? How often do you find that there's an interference in your journey from all kinds of things, circumstances, thoughts, temptations, and who knows what else? The apostle Paul identifies with you. As an apostle, he had his own journey of overcoming. He shared it with us when he confessed that sometimes he did the very things he didn't want to do.

When he says, *"If then I do those things **that I would not do**,"* Paul is basically saying, "If I practice unforgiveness, it overtakes me. I hate it. I know I should always forgive, but for some reason I find myself holding grudges and records of wrongs and practicing unforgiveness. I hate unforgiveness, but I can't stop myself from *practicing* unforgiveness." It is the same as saying that the law of God—the law of forgiveness—is evil, and the law of unforgiveness is good. So, these two laws are battling inside you. The law and nature of God brings you health. The law of sin and nature of Satan brings you disease. The question for you to consider is this: Which law are you being influenced by today?

THE SNARE OF THE ENEMY

Over thirty years ago, when I asked the Lord why I didn't see more healing in my ministry as a pastor, God led me to 2 Timothy 2:24–26:

> *And the servant of the Lord must not strive, must be gentle unto all men, patient, apt to teach in meekness instructing those that oppose themselves; if God peradventure will give them repentance to the acknowledging of the truth; and that they may recover themselves **out of the snare of the devil, who are taken captive by him at his will.***

Whoa, what? *"Recover themselves out of the snare of the devil"* and *"who are taken captive by him at his will!"* "Lord," I prayed, "this letter is written to Christians; how can this be happening?" My eyes were opened when I realized what Paul was saying. His words reveal that there can be something in a Christian's life that gives the devil a legal right to take them captive, to steal their blessings, and to put disease on them. I want to remind you that not all disease comes to people in this way. Not every disease has a spiritual root of sin, but I have found without question that a large portion of the chronic diseases that I have confronted have a spiritual root.

Jesus linked the law of sin and healing more than once in the New Testament. When He met the paralyzed man lying beside the pool of Bethsaida, Jesus healed the man by telling him to take up his bed and walk. Hours later, they met again in the temple. This time, Jesus told that same man that now that he was healed, he should go and sin no more, or something much worse would happen to him. *"Afterward Jesus findeth him in the temple, and said unto him, Behold, thou art made whole: sin no more, lest a worse thing come unto thee"* (John 5:14). Disease had come to this man through the law of sin; Jesus encouraged him to sin no more.

Other times, Jesus used both the phrases "you are healed" and "your sins are forgiven" when He healed someone. Matthew 9:1–5 and in Mark 2:5–10 record the same healing. *"And, behold, they brought to him a man sick of the palsy, lying on a bed: and Jesus seeing their faith said unto the sick of the palsy; Son, be of good cheer; thy sins be forgiven thee"* (Matthew 9:2). And the man was healed; he got up and walked. As we can see from the Scriptures, there can definitely be a connection between sickness and the law of sin in our lives.

REPENTANCE IS NOT A BAD WORD

> *That God peradventure will give them **repentance** to the acknowledging of the truth that they may **recover themselves from the snare of the devil**, who are taken captive by him at his will.* (2 Timothy 2:25–26)

Paul shared this Word with us because when we know the truth of God's law, of God's true nature, it brings us to *repentance*. Now, repentance is not a bad word. It doesn't mean that you are not a Christian or that you are an evil person. Paul was speaking to New Testament believers when he talked about this repentance. Can you imagine going to the Father, the Lord of creation, and saying, "Dad, I'm sorry. I come to You in Jesus's name, Father. I yielded to Satan's law of sin. I've been following it, but I hate it. I don't want to do it anymore. As it says in Your Word, it's not good for me. I come to You to take responsibility for my sin, and I repent to You for allowing it to control my life. Will You please forgive me?"

Is that hard? Oftentimes, we need to deal with sin and spiritual issues that are affecting our hearts before our healing can occur. That is a prescription directly from heaven. No health insurance is needed, and it may save you from incurable diseases! Folks, you can do a lot to prevent disease in your life. Read these truths carefully and embrace them. We're so busy chasing symptoms and disease profiles that we don't take into account why we got sick in the first place.

We experience *repentance* from our sins when we first turn to God to acknowledge Jesus Christ's death and resurrection on our behalf. That is our *salvation*. Now, it would be great if, once we became Christians, we never sinned again. But that isn't what happens. Thank God that even when we do sin, and then confess it to God, He is always gracious to forgive us. *"If we say that we have no sin, we deceive ourselves, and the truth is not in us. If we confess our sins, he is faithful and just to forgive us our sins, and to cleanse us from all unrighteousness"* (1 John 1:8–9).

Sanctification also plays an important role in our becoming free from disease. As Christians, we need further repentance for things in our lives that aren't of God. That is our *sanctification.* Sanctification is a lifelong process for the Christian where, through the glories and trials of life, and through our obedience to Him, we learn to walk in the newness of life. *"That like as Christ was raised up from the dead by the glory of the Father, even so we also should walk in newness of life"* (Romans 6:4). Sanctification is God's plan for us. Our part is to embrace His truth, repent of any part of the law of sin, and allow Him to transform us into His image.

IT'S CONVICTION, NOT CONDEMNATION!

Please don't react to God's truth about sin in your life by condemning yourself. The Holy Spirit reveals our sins to us in order to bring repentance and freedom, not to condemn us! His conviction helps us recognize our sin so that we can repent and walk in the freedom of Jesus Christ. *"There is therefore now no condemnation to them which are in Christ Jesus, who walk not after the flesh, but after the Spirit"* (Romans 8:1). This is all the process of our sanctification, of our being changed as we grow in Him.

Our greatest encouragement is that the Holy Spirit is there to help us through the whole sanctification process. The Bible tells us, *"But we all, with open face beholding as in a glass the glory of the Lord, are changed into the same image from glory to glory, even as by the Spirit of the Lord"* (2 Corinthians 3:18). The words *"are changed into the same image"* are in the present progressive tense. That means that being changed into Christ's image is an ongoing process; we become more like Christ as we walk out our sanctification throughout our lives.

I do want you to understand that God is not going to live your life for you. That is why God gives you the responsibility of believing the truth of the Word when it comes to the battle with the law of sin. You must take ownership in this victory; you must activate; you must decide to wake up, be an overcomer, and face the things from the enemy in your life and defeat them in Jesus's name. Embrace the process of sanctification from God so that you can walk in the freedom of Jesus Christ!

UNFORGIVENESS AND DISEASE

Nearly twenty years ago, *Newsweek* magazine featured an article that startled the scientific community.[3] Research was uncovered that forgiveness and unforgiveness affect human health. When medical science discovered this truth, they declared that unforgiveness was a disease. They named it a disease because they recognized its effect on the human body. However, that's not what the Bible calls it. The Bible calls unforgiveness sin.

Our biggest problem in overcoming disease is that people want to be healed without getting rid of the sins that are at the root of the disease. One of the greatest blocks to healing is the sin of unforgiveness. If you embrace unforgiveness, you are following the law of sin. Unforgiveness is one of the spiritual roots of disease. Don't hold on to the wrongs committed by others. Be a doer of the Word. Be a forgiver.

3. Jerry Adler, "Live and Let Live," *Newsweek*, October 3, 2004, https://www.newsweek.com/forgive-and-let-live-129513.

I want to share with you the power of repentance from unforgiveness in the healing of disease. Some years ago, I had the opportunity to minister to a fifty-year-old pastor's wife who was diagnosed with stage four breast cancer. It had metastasized, and the doctors gave her no hope for survival. She'd been prayed for by her husband and the elders of the church, but there was no change. Her doctor, who was also a member of her church, heard about my work with the spiritual roots of disease and said to her, "Maybe you should call Pastor Wright."

Her husband called me, and then his wife got on the phone. What happened next was a very frank conversation. This dear woman was looking for another prayer for a supernatural healing, but I was looking for the spiritual root of her disease so that she could be healed and set free. I told her, "You have already been prayed for by many. We need to follow the Word of God concerning the law of sin and disease." As we talked about the battle with the law of sin, she began to search her heart. Finally, I asked her, "Do you have any unforgiveness or bitterness against another woman?" Why did I ask that question? Because in my three-decade journey of fighting disease, a high percentage of case histories have revealed that a woman who gets breast cancer has bitterness and unforgiveness in her life, often against another woman.

After my question, this woman became very quiet. Then she admitted, "Yes, I do." I was excited, even though I didn't let it show, because I knew we were moving in the right direction. James 5:16 says, *"Confess your faults one to another, and pray one for another, that ye may be healed."* I knew that her healing required confession, repentance, and forgiveness.

TAKE RESPONSIBILITY FOR YOUR LIFE

I asked this woman what she thought she should do next. "I think I need to repent to the Father." She thought again, and then she said, "Well, I think what I need to do is not just confess to the Father. I need to contact this woman, confess to her that I've had this bitterness, and ask her to forgive me." She would call her to say, "I've had this unforgiveness. I hate it. It is sin in my life. I ask you to forgive me." I knew that when she confessed to the Father and also asked for this woman's forgiveness, she would be forgiven. *"For if ye forgive men their trespasses, your heavenly Father will also forgive you"* (Matthew 6:14). Of course, the Scripture goes on to say, *"But if ye forgive not men their trespasses, neither will your Father forgive your trespasses"* (verse 15). We can't forget that. We must forgive!

Forgiving others is one of the major keys to receiving from God. This pastor's wife made the life-changing decision to take responsibility for her unforgiveness against this other woman. She approached her with a pure heart of conviction to forgive her and to ask for her forgiveness. Even though the cancer was metastasized, I knew the power of the cross would break the power of the enemy over her.

I never heard from her again. However, a few months later, I received a book in the mail entitled *The Biblical Guide to Alternative Medicine*, autographed by the author, Dr. Michael Jacobson. Dr. Jacobson was the woman's medical doctor who attended their church and had counseled her to call me. When I read his book, I discovered that the pastor's wife had received a complete healing from her cancer! God was faithful to His Word!

How did her healing occur? I just brought the truth; she had to be obedient and do the rest. Her heart was opened and submitted to God by confessing and repenting of her sin toward another. She became a doer of the Word and not just a hearer. *"But be ye doers of the word, and not hearers only, deceiving your own selves"* (James 1:22). Why become a doer of the Word? So that we no longer *deceive ourselves,* and we can recover ourselves from the snare of the devil!

WHY WOULD YOU TAKE THEIR SIN?

I have already stated that 20 percent of chronic diseases do not have a spiritual root. However, if you have a disease, wouldn't you want to search the Scriptures and also search your heart? Wouldn't you go to the Lord with this request from Psalm 139, *"Search me, O God, and know my heart: try me, and know my thoughts: and see if there be any wicked way in me, and lead me in the way everlasting"* (Psalm 139:23–24)? When you think of someone in particular, do you feel a high-octane *ping* go off deep inside of you? Consider that you may be holding unforgiveness or resentment in your heart toward that person. If what is keeping you from your healing is the law of sin, which is the opposite of the Word of God, don't you want to repent of it and move on to a life of wholeness and health? Confess it before the Lord and be free.

If you decide to follow the law of sin, instead, and hold a record of wrongs against another person, it will likely produce a disease in your body. That's true even though that person sinned against you—wronged you, betrayed you. It was their sin. But because of your agreement with a spirit of bitterness, you now have a disease.

I need to ask you a very serious question. I don't want you to forget this question as long as you live because your life may depend on it. *Why would you take the sins of another person into your body?*

Jesus took that sin so that you don't have to. He forgave them. He went to the cross, and as He hung there dying, He was asking His Father to forgive the very person that you won't forgive today. If you take another person's failure against you into your heart and into your body, you can expect trouble to come on you in your lifetime. Be kind to yourself and forgive them. Release them, get your heart right with God, and then keep moving on in freedom. You will still have the memory, but God will heal the pain. The kindest thing you can do for yourself is to forgive others.

DON'T BE EASY PICKINGS FOR SATAN!

Feelings can be a source of temptation that comes from Satan's kingdom. That's what happened to Adam and Eve. They had feelings and thoughts. They embraced them. Then, they followed them. Do you think you're not easy pickings for Satan's temptation? Please don't think that you aren't tempted by the law of sin, or that you are stronger than Paul in overcoming temptation! What about Peter? At the Last Supper, Peter basically said to Jesus, "Tonight I will die this death with You." The Lord looked at him over a communion table and answered, "Peter, tonight, you will deny Me three times!" (See, for example, Luke 22:31–34.)

It's clear to see there is a war going on within. God defeated Satan, but Satan still roams this earth like a roaring lion seeking whom he might devour. *"Be sober, be vigilant; because your adversary the devil, as a roaring lion, walketh about, seeking whom he may devour"* (1 Peter 5:8). God desires to free us through His Word and His Holy Spirit, but the enemy wants to capture us through his lies and deceptions. The choice is yours. Who do you want to be your master?

THE POWER OF GRACE AND MERCY

Please don't be discouraged or afraid of the battle we must face between the law of sin and the law of God. God is showing us truth so that He can make us free. *"If the Son therefore shall make you free, ye shall be free indeed"* (John 8:36). When Paul looked at the critical battle in his own life, he cried out, "Who will save me?" His answer is the same as our answer today! *"O wretched man that I am! who shall deliver me from the body of this death? **I thank God through Jesus Christ our Lord**"* (Romans 7:24–25). Our victory in this battle comes from the Lord Jesus Christ!

Jesus's life, death, and resurrection brought us the Father's grace and mercy. God's grace gives us the power to make the right choices. God's grace is teaching us the things we need to know as children of God, and the Holy Spirit is giving us the power to defeat the influence of Satan and the law of sin in our lives. Grace's companion is mercy. Mercy is the amount of time God gives us to figure out what He is saying to us through His

Word and through His Spirit. Thank God that we are living in the dispensation of His grace and mercy!

RESPONDING TO GOD IN LOVE

Through Jesus Christ, God has removed the power of the law and given us the opportunity for our heart to respond to Him, not out of fear, not because of legalism, but because He loves us and we love Him. You can go and sin no more and allow the Lord to renew you in His grace and mercy. It's a daily journey for each of us.

Do not open your life to Satan's lies. Sometimes we fall into his deception and don't even realize it. Keep your spiritual eyes open to the truth of God's Word. You don't have to obey unforgiveness. You don't have to obey anger. You don't have to obey fear. You don't have to obey lust. You don't have to obey shame. You don't have to obey anything that's not God's nature. When having done all to stand, just stand, man or woman of God. Just stand! Let the enemy know your resolve. *"Neither yield ye your members as instruments of unrighteousness unto sin but yield yourselves unto God as those that are alive from the dead and your members as instruments of righteousness unto God"* (Romans 6:13). You must make this decision.

Will you appropriate the freedom the Father has purchased for you through the blood of His Son? Will you choose to embrace the nature and the law of God or the law of sin? Will you choose forgiveness, love, and peace—or will you choose unforgiveness, bitterness, hatred, fear, and anxiety? God has given you a choice. Choose life.

Five

WHO CONTROLS OUR THOUGHTS?

Where do our thoughts come from? Is everything we think from ourselves? For Christians, some of our thoughts are from the Holy Spirit. Some of our thoughts are our own. Some of our thoughts are also from the enemy—Satan. Your body is a *responder* to who you are in thought. It's referred to as the mind-body connection. It's not anything new to a believer. God already told us, *"As a man thinketh in his heart, so is he"* (Proverbs 23:7). God knew what He was talking about! It is a biological truth that the things we think about and dwell on actually become part of who we are. We will never get to the spiritual roots of disease if we don't first understand the biology of how our minds affect our bodies.

This is not a new concept in the medical field, either. Science discovered the mind-body connection long ago. This connection is taught in all medical training centers. What is *not taught* is the *spirit*-mind (soul)-body connection. As a result, not many people understand that it is not just a mind-body connection, but that our spirits are involved as well—it's a *spirit-soul-body* connection.

I'm emphasizing again that you must understand this truth in order to move on to freedom from disease.

We acquire the mind of Christ by meditating on His Word, thinking as He thinks, and embracing God's ways and His nature. We're supposed to be moving forward in God's Word, not shrinking in truth and knowledge. You need to know how to acquire the mind of Christ because your mind plays a crucial role in the spiritual roots of disease. You need to understand that not all of our thoughts come from ourselves. Some of them come from our enemy. And those thoughts bring the roots of disease with them.

THE ORIGIN OF OUR THOUGHTS

We have already established that God is a spirit, the enemy is a spirit, and you are a spirit, with a soul and a body. God communicates with us spirit to spirit. Unfortunately, so does the enemy. You receive thoughts at the spirit level—within you—and record them at the soul level, in your mind and emotions. The important thing to understand about your thoughts is that they might not be yours! They could come from you, from the Holy Spirit, or from Satan's kingdom. That is why it is vital for your health that you understand that your thoughts have different origins.

When a thought passes through our mind, we may naturally assume that it comes from us. However, it might have been given to us by an invisible enemy from an invisible kingdom who will then make it sound just like us by "speaking" in the first person. Satan tempts us with negative thoughts; he plants the thoughts, repeats the thoughts, and we are deceived into accepting them as our own. We embrace them and take ownership of them. Then, the enemy uses those same thoughts to control us spiritually, psychologically, and biologically. Those thoughts are what the Bible calls temptations.

TEMPTATION TRAINS YOU

We are very aware that what the Bible calls temptation, the world has redefined as mere negative emotions or psychological defects. They insist it's just emotional issues rather than a spiritual problem. But that's not what Jesus taught. Jesus taught it was a spiritual problem. Too many Christians are woefully ignorant about temptation. They act like temptation and sin don't exist anymore. The church might dismiss temptation, or they may call it a human problem; some may even go into an altered state of consciousness through prescription drugs to avoid it. But "out of sight, out of mind" is not a spiritual principle! God doesn't want you to be mindless. He wants you to be awake to the truth and to be redeemed from the lies!

Temptation comes to us in thoughts and feelings. Obviously, the thoughts that come to you every day are not always good ones. You might be thinking, "Well, I just wish I wouldn't have these negative, bad thoughts." Unfortunately, none of us is immune to temptation. Not even Jesus was immune to temptation even though He never sinned. You are not immune to the influence of a spirit world that wants to get you to listen. Wake up! You need to understand the Word of God well enough to know what is of God and what isn't. Then you can embrace the truth.

Temptation comes to train you. Be careful what you listen to and what you watch. The enemy wants you to listen to him. He wants to use thoughts and temptations to train you in the law of sin, to train you to be sick. You need to check those thoughts against the Word of God. When the enemy comes to attack you, you need to quit blaming yourself for thoughts that aren't even yours. You've embraced thoughts and feelings like Adam and Eve did. You've been carrying them most of your lifetime. Why do that? Be kind to yourself.

SHORT-TERM AND LONG-TERM MEMORY

Let's look closely at how our mind (soul) is involved in this spirit-soul-body connection. You have an active brain with thoughts popping up all over the place, along with feelings and emotions. Your brain is a miraculous processor for these things. The basics of life depend on your thinking. Your mind is continually dwelling on something—whether good or bad. If you're not meditating on the Word of God, you're meditating on something else.

Initially, what we perceive all around us—what we experience during our day—is stored in our short-term memory. What we have in our short-term memory will be forgotten if it is not moved into our long-term memory. For this to happen, a biological event must take place in our brain called *protein synthesis*. The process, which involves our RNA, is essential for this memory transaction to occur. Once the thought is in long-term memory, we can remember it and recall it. And the more often we recall or dwell on the thought or experience, the more permanent it becomes in our brains.

Listen carefully. After time, *that thought becomes permanently part of your soul.* It becomes a part of your mind, part of your emotions, part of your personality—part *of your biology.* Good thoughts become permanently a part of your biology. The Word of God becomes permanently a part of your biology. And sinful thoughts become a permanent part of your biology, as well. They become part of the way you think and act. For that reason, both God and Satan want their ways to be stored in your long-term memory.

God uses this process that He created in us to build long-term memory when we meditate on His Word, when we meditate on the truths of His love for us. But so does the enemy when we meditate on his lies—things like, "The Bible is outdated; you don't have to follow it." "You're a worthless loser." "You fail at everything you do." You need to hear something six times in order to retain 25 percent of it in your long-term memory. I know that when the enemy comes along, he does not give you a thought only six times. He may give you that thought every day for years on end because he wants to program you to have a disorder or disease. You are in his sights because of a lack of understanding of Satan's devices—his plans and his schemes.

Please understand that this is a journey from the inside out. God wants to influence us from within, by His Spirit and by His Word. The kingdom of darkness wants to influence us from within as well. God speaks to you from within to train you in His nature and righteousness, while the enemy speaks to you from within to train you in death and destruction. Satan has been training the human race in the law of sin since the time of Adam and Eve.

MEDITATE ON GOD'S WORD

In order to allow the Word of God to become a part of your biology, to become flesh of your flesh, you must meditate on it. How often does God say to meditate on the Word? Day and night. *"Blessed is the man that walketh not in the counsel of the ungodly, nor standeth in the way of sinners, nor sitteth in the seat of the scornful. But his delight is in the law of the LORD; and in his law doth he meditate* ***day and night***" (Psalm 1:1–2).

God knows that if you meditate on His Word, it will become a permanent part of you. In this way, God has given us *the antidote to the law of sin*. If you do not have this antidote, all you have is the law of sin without the spiritual power to defeat it. You can go on an antidepressant to try to suppress bad thoughts and temptations, but it will not help you change your mindset. What will help you change your mindset is if you read and apply God's Word, which is life and truth, and begin the process of coming out of disease and into freedom! (You can begin to renew your mind while still on the medication. Please do not stop your medicine without the supervision of your doctor.)

Satan is banking on your being so unfamiliar with the truth of God's Word that he can successfully tempt you with the law of sin. He can control your thinking and then blame you, as if the thought behind it were original to you. So, you have the bad thought and the guilt of it, all from his hands. We can be so easily duped by the enemy!

TAKE THOSE THOUGHTS CAPTIVE!

Thankfully, we serve a God of grace and mercy! He is not going to leave us defenseless against Satan's onslaught of thoughts and temptations. Jesus understands our battle against the enemy because He battled him, as well. You know your personal battles. What are you going to do with the thoughts that come from the enemy and compete with the Word of God? You're going to use the spiritual weapons of warfare that God has given you! You're going to take those thoughts captive and cast them down as evil imaginations. *"For the weapons of our warfare are not carnal, but mighty through God to the pulling down of strong holds; **casting down** imaginations, and every high thing that exalteth itself against the knowledge of God, and **bringing into captivity every thought** to the obedience of Christ"* (2 Corinthians 10:5).

What does it mean to "bring every thought into captivity"? It means considering the origin of every thought you have, every feeling, every emotion, every picture, everything that surges through your spirit and mind. Those feelings, apprehensions, and thoughts can cause biological manifestations, such as disease and disorders in your body. You are going to test those thoughts against the Word of God. Are they truth or a trap from the enemy? Then you are going to embrace the truth and not the lie.

Now, I don't want you to think that I am advocating a "mind over matter philosophy." This is not you accomplishing all this in your own strength alone. This is the power of the Word of God and the Holy Spirit enabling you to do what the Word directs you to do! Casting down false imaginations is a powerful weapon that God has given us to fight the enemy. Why would you ignore His help? It's like a soldier going into battle and leaving his rifle behind. Cast down those imaginations and anything that doesn't measure up to the knowledge of God.

Meditating on the Word of God means that you read it, memorize it, think about it often, and embrace it as being truth in your life. You will recognize the source of your thoughts by how they measure against those Scriptures, and you will reject any thoughts that do not line up with God's Word. Take those thoughts captive to the obedience of Jesus Christ and kick them to the curb—for good!

YOU NEED SPIRITUAL DISCERNMENT

When false thoughts come to you claiming that you are not loved by God, or God has rejected you, take hold of those thoughts and ask yourself, "Where did these thoughts come from? Did they originate from the Word of God?" No, they didn't, because God's Word says that if we are believers, God dwells in us and loves us, and nothing shall be able to separate us from His love. *"God is love; and he that dwelleth in love dwelleth in God, and God in him"* (1 John 4:16). *"For I am convinced that neither death nor life, neither angels nor demons...nor anything else in all creation, will be able to separate us from **the love of God** that is in Christ Jesus our Lord"* (Romans 8:38–39).

We all need spiritual discernment. Spiritual discernment requires examining the origin of thought with the guidance of the Holy Spirit. If fear comes to tempt you—whether fear of man, fear of rejection, fear of failure, fear of death, or fear of something else—you can go directly to the Word of God and declare, "That's not from God. According to His Word, God has not given me the spirit of fear! *'God hath not given us the spirit of fear; but of power, and of love, and of a sound mind'* (2 Timothy 1:7). I'm not listening to those lies any longer!" That is how you take hold of those thoughts and cast them down as imaginations!

The lies from the enemy that you once meditated on will become a diminished part of your persona because you're not focusing on them any longer. It will become easier and easier to cast down a lying thought because you recognize what it is, you cast it down, and you move on. That is how you become an overcomer!

No one can do this for you. You must learn to embrace the Word of God for yourself. God will be there to encourage you by His Holy Spirit, but you have to choose to do this. Don't wallow in self-pity or engage in excessive self-talk about your sickness and disease. Don't make excuses. The Holy Spirit lives within you and gives you the strength and the power to make these choices. Take those thoughts captive to the obedience of Jesus Christ. Do it.

RENEWING YOUR MIND

Romans 12:2 says, *"Be not conformed to this world: but be ye transformed by the renewing of your mind."*

The Bible talks about renewing our minds, which is also why God tells us to meditate on His Word day and night. Your mind is renewed, or cleansed, from Satan's lies and thought patterns by being washed with the water of the Word. *"That he might sanctify and cleanse it with the washing of water by the word"* (Ephesians 5:26). This cleansed mind now confronts your bad thinking and teaches you how to think righteously. You can learn how God wants you to think and apply it to your life. If you have fear, anxiety, or stress, this is the process of getting free. This is how we become spiritual people in how we think, speak, and act. I ask God our Father to join you in your journey so that you can be conformed into His image.

As painful as it can be for people to face the truth about hidden things in their lives, at Be in Health, it is our calling to present that truth and compel Christians to face their fears, anxieties, and sins. Don't be afraid. The renewing of our minds must happen for us to have victory. As a result of our minds being renewed in God's Word, we will be delivered from the diseases that afflict the rest of the world. God gave us the key in Romans 12:1–2:

> *I beseech you therefore, brethren, by the mercies of God, that ye present your bodies a living sacrifice, holy, acceptable unto God, which is your reasonable service. And be not conformed to this world: but be ye transformed by the renewing of your mind, that ye may prove what is that good, and acceptable, and perfect, will of God.*

Listen to God! Do not listen to the world!

Six

THE PATHWAY OF DISEASE

Bless the LORD...who forgiveth all thine iniquities;
who healeth all thy diseases.
—Psalm 103:2–3

I had some personal experiences with the spirit-soul-body connection very early in my ministry. I was a young pastor in my first church. It was a storefront church in Florida, and we were having prayer meetings every Monday night. During one prayer meeting, a young woman came into the church. Her husband was in the car, and he was overcome with muscle spasms, shaking and falling to the floor.

I ran out to the sidewalk and yanked open the passenger door of the car. Her husband was half in the seat and half on the floor, shaking violently. It was so startling that the first thing that came out of my mouth was, "Whoa!" I thought, "What are you going to do with that?" "Call 9-1-1" was the logical answer. But

I stopped first to pray, saying, "Father, I haven't the foggiest idea what's going on, but You do."

I was a pre-med student in college, so I had some knowledge of the human body. One word jumped into my mind as soon as I began praying: *hypothalamus*. I found myself praying this: "I take authority over the spirit of fear that's giving signals to the hypothalamus to produce this involuntary muscle spasm. I command the spirit of fear to be gone, and the hypothalamus to not take any more information from that spirit of fear. Central nervous system, be at peace; muscle spasms, stop now, in Jesus's name." And just like that, it stopped. Her husband sat back up on that passenger seat, and she drove him home. We went back into the prayer meeting in awe of what God had just done.

LAUNCHING A JOURNEY

I was shocked to realize that I had spoken accurately to the evil spirit that had taken over this man's mind with feelings and thoughts that caused him to become fearful. This fear had triggered the hypothalamus gland to begin producing neurological signals causing the involuntary muscle spasms that had him on the floor of his car. I learned a never-forgotten lesson that night: God has given us a connection between the spirit, the soul, and the body.

That night I launched out on a thirty-plus-year journey to study the connection between thought and physiology. The result of those studies are tens of thousands of people worldwide who now have the knowledge for their freedom from disease. It's my desire to pass this knowledge on to you, as well. Some of the details are a little technical, but please keep tracking with me. It is for your life and health.

God has created the human body with a plan for your health. You need to understand how your body is constructed—as well as how that plan is thwarted by the decisions you make in your thought life. God has given you an amazing human body with many highly functioning systems. You have a brain, a nervous system, a cardiovascular system, heart rhythm, skin, hair, eyes, ears, and nose. You have a skeletal form, muscles, kidneys, bone marrow, blood vessels, and lymph glands. You have your liver, lungs, intestines, urinary tract, and endocrine system, including important glands like the amygdalae and hypothalamus glands. This is you. This is what you are on the inside. You are a creative miracle. And all of these systems are highly responsive and regulated by a process that *originates in your brain*.

YOUR BRAIN AND YOUR NERVOUS SYSTEM

There are two parts to your nervous system. First, the *voluntary* nervous system which gives you voluntary control of your body movements. You can tell your arm to rise up and scratch your head when you want to. Second, you have the *involuntary*, or *sympathetic*, nervous system, which God created so that your heart would pump and you could breathe without thinking about it; your digestive organs work, passing food through your body without you giving it another thought. However, if you have a long-term memory full of thoughts that oppose God's Word, your brain can interfere with both the voluntary and the involuntary nervous system, causing them to function improperly; that is what I call the *dis*-ease of function. *Dis*-ease is exactly what it sounds like—the lack of *ease* or health within your spirit and your body's systems.

Now, stay with me here as we go a little further. Look at Chart 1. We are looking at the brain. Your limbic system is the part of the brain that deals with your emotions and your memory. There are four main parts in the limbic system, but to understand the roots of disease, I want to focus on two in particular: the *amygdala* and the *hypothalamus* glands.

Tracking Fear in the Brain

3. ASSOCIATION CORTEX
Separates threats from false alarms. Was that loud noise a gunshot or just a car backfiring?

HYPOTHALAMUS

1. THALAMUS
Routes information from the eyes and ears to other parts of the brain for processing.

4. HIPPOCAMPUS
Helps evaluate threats by placing them in context of previous experiences. A frightening noise heard in a place you consider safe is less likely to scare you.

5. PREFRONTAL CORTEX
Reins in the amygdala if an initial threat is deemed insignificant.

2. AMYGDALA
The brain's rapid response system. Sends the body into high alert if triggered.

Chart 1

The amygdalae are two almond-shaped glands near the frontal lobe area of your brain. Each is a cluster of nerve cells that are responsible for what we call the "fight-or-flight" reaction to emergency situations, stress, and fear. The amygdalae also play a vital role in storing our long-term memories. The amygdalae and the hypothalamus are involved in our deeply felt emotions, whether negative (such as panic, anger, fear) or positive (such as love, laughter, joy).

THE HYPOTHALAMUS: A SMALL GLAND WITH A BIG JOB

How does this affect our bodies in relation to disease? I want to explain to you the importance of the pea-sized gland called the hypothalamus. It's very significant in our understanding of the spiritual roots of disease. We are going to expose the specific pathway that Satan uses to bring disease to mankind.

Let's look at Chart 2 and see what the hypothalamus gland controls. Your endocrine system is a chemical messenger system that involves several important glands in your body, including the pituitary gland, the adrenal glands, and the hypothalamus gland. These glands secrete hormones that keep your body balanced and working smoothly. Of these glands, the *hypothalamus* is considered the brain, or the *control center*, of the entire endocrine system. It is a small but vital gland in the center of your brain.

The main role of the hypothalamus is to keep your body in *homeostasis*, which means in a healthy body balance. It regulates the other glands, telling them when they should secrete the hormones that are necessary *for every system* in your body to

Endocrine System

Chart 2

remain in homeostasis, or in a healthy balance. Your body works continually to maintain this balance because without it, you will develop a disorder or disease.

THE MASTER CONTROL

As the master control, the hypothalamus regulates many bodily activities: your body temperature, thirst, appetite and weight control, emotions, sleep cycles, sex drive, childbirth, blood pressure and heart rate, production of digestive juices, and balancing of bodily fluids. It activates your thyroid, which, in turn, affects your metabolism, energy levels, and developmental growth. It stirs the pituitary gland to release the growth hormones we all need.

The hypothalamus is working continually, controlling the release of hormones from the other endocrine glands to maintain homeostasis in all of these systems. For example, if the hypothalamus receives a message that your body temperature is too high, it will trigger the appropriate gland to produce sweat. If it receives the message that your body temperature is too low, it will create heat by shivering. As a result, unless you are sick, your body maintains something close to 98.6 degrees Fahrenheit at all times. It's an astounding amount of work for a small gland most people have never heard of before!

Since the hypothalamus regulates your heart rate, the actual contraction of your heart muscles, and the movement of food through the digestive system, serious problems occur when it is not functioning normally. An interference with the hypothalamus in the function of your cardiovascular system can cause high blood pressure and heart attacks. In the gastrointestinal system, this interference can result in such things as ulcerative colitis, irritable bowel syndrome, diarrhea, vomiting, and nausea.

WHAT YOU MEDITATE ON REGULATES THE HYPOTHALAMUS

Our main focus here is that the hypothalamus is also the center of the spirit-soul-body connection for disease that we have been discussing. This is so important for you to understand. Take a look at Chart 1 again. The cerebral cortex covers the largest part of the brain. It's how we process information, our thinking, language comprehension, problem solving, and—most important for this study—our long-term memory. When you are meditating on thoughts of fear, anxiety, bitterness, anger, self-hatred, or shame, the amygdalae receive and interpret those strong negative emotions and thoughts as a threat. The rest of the limbic system kicks into survival mode, and the hypothalamus gland responds.

The hypothalamus receives these negative messages from your thoughts and may become overwhelmed. The result may be hypo- or hyperactivity in the endocrine system, neurological misfiring in your brain, or neurotransmitter imbalance. Your constant negative thoughts—and the evil spirits behind them—have disrupted the proper working of the hypothalamus gland, and a hypothalamus gland that is not at peace can lead to diseases and disorders in any part of your body.

A lack of homeostasis can affect the gastrointestinal system, create sexual disorders (impotence and frigidity), cause skin diseases (eczema, neurodermatitis, acne, etc.), and lead to diabetes and amenorrhea, fatigue and lethargy, overeating, depression, and insomnia. In addition, it can lead to coronary artery disease, hypertension/disturbance of heart rhythm, tension, headaches, muscle contractions, back aches, rheumatoid arthritis, related inflammatory diseases, asthma, hay fever, and immunosuppressant autoimmune disease. All these conditions stem from a dysfunction with the hypothalamus gland, creating a lack of homeostasis or balance in your body.

Medical science agrees with the role of the hypothalamus in responding to our emotions. Scientists agree that our minds—through strong negative thoughts and emotions—can create an imbalance of homeostasis. As I assured you earlier, I am not an enemy of science. Look at the information it has provided for our understanding of the physical function of the brain and the hypothalamus gland. The medical community has concluded:

"According to the mind-body or biopsychosocial paradigm, which supersedes the older biomedical model, there is no real division between mind and body because of networks of communication that exist between the brain and neurological, endocrine and immune systems," said Oakley Ray, Professor Emeritus of Psychology, Psychiatry and Pharmacology at Vanderbilt University (Nashville, TN, USA).[4]

Science confirms that there is a direct correspondence between anxiety and palpitations.[5] There is a direct correspondence between hostility and coronary artery thrombosis.[6] There is also a direct connection between shame and irritable bowel syndrome.[7]

---

4. Brower, "Mind-Body Research Moves Toward the Mainstream."
5. Peter Tyrer and David Baldwin, "Generalised Anxiety Disorder," *Lancet* 368 (2006): 2156–66, https://www.sciencedirect.com/science/article/abs/pii/S0140673606698656.
6. Daichi Shimbo et al., "Hostility and Platelet Reactivity in Individuals Without a History of Cardiovascular Disease Events," *Psychosomatic Medicine* 71 (2009): 741–7, https://journals.lww.com/psychosomaticmedicine/Abstract/2009/09000/Hostility_and_Platelet_Reactivity_in_Individuals.7.aspx.
7. Douglas A. Drossman et al., "A Focus Group Assessment of Patient Perspectives on Irritable Bowel Syndrome and Illness Severity," *Digestive Diseases and Sciences* 54 (2009): 1532–41, https://pubmed.ncbi.nlm.nih.gov/19337833/.

THE HYPOTHALAMUS IS THE PATHWAY THE ENEMY USES

Now, how is our spirit-man involved in this connection between the mind, the hypothalamus gland, and disease? Remember, the soul (the mind and emotions) is the bridge between the spirit world and the physical world. God uses the hypothalamus gland to maintain a *balance* of homeostasis in our bodies. The devil uses it to create an *imbalance* of homeostasis. All of this is done through our thoughts and emotions.

If the hypothalamus can be triggered into dysfunction through temptations—and if a lack of homeostasis can cause disease—then the enemy has a clear pathway to bring disease into our lives, doesn't he? The hypothalamus gland is the enemy's entryway to create many diseases in our bodies. Let's walk through this whole process again. Here is the pathway:

Step One: The enemy tempts you with thoughts that oppose the Word of God—thoughts of unrighteousness, such as unforgiveness, bitterness, self-hatred, greed, envy, jealousy, anger, hostility, fear, stress, and anxiety. These are part of the law of sin.

Step Two: If you embrace those unrighteous thoughts and emotions as your own and meditate regularly on them instead of on the Word of God, they become a part of your long-term memory and a part of your actual biology.

Step Three: These elevated negative thoughts and emotions, and the evil spirits behind them, are then communicated from your amygdalae glands and the cerebral cortex to the hypothalamus gland. The hypothalamus then triggers the wrong signals (hormones, etc.) to other vital glands throughout your body.

Now, this isn't a onetime occurrence. It can happen to you day after day, year after year, even beginning in childhood. As a result, your homeostasis becomes unbalanced, and you find yourself combating serious diseases possibly including heart disease, cancer, autoimmune diseases, diabetes, and many more.

For each disease, there is a *door point*, a place where the spirit of infirmity can come in and wreak havoc. The enemy can use thoughts of fear, bitterness, shame, and many other things to wear down the immune system. From that door point, the enemy enters with the spirit of infirmity to bring you disease. "*And he was teaching in one of the synagogues on the sabbath. And, behold, there was a woman which had a spirit of infirmity eighteen years, and was bowed together, and could in no wise lift up herself. And when Jesus saw her, he called her to him, and said unto her, Woman, thou art loosed from thine infirmity. And he laid his hands on her: and immediately she was made straight, and glorified God*" (Luke 13:10–13).

What a devious plan of the enemy! Think about it. The little hypothalamus gland is the only gland that Satan and his spirit of infirmity need to move you in the direction of disease! Instead of our body functioning as God intended, we have *dis*-ease of function. If that *dis*-ease continues, it may transform into a full-blown disorder or disease. Satan understands how the human body functions. The enemy just needs that one gland to set this whole mess in motion. He understands what he needs to do to send you into imbalance and to wreak havoc with your health. He is good at it, but, thankfully, God is so much bigger! That is why we are laying out this knowledge so that you will know how to fight Satan's plan of disease for your life.

I want you to have the victory over the enemy's plan for you! We are intense about this because your life and health are at stake. At Be in Health, we have a God-given zeal to get this message out to as many people as possible. Church, it's time to wake up! Salvation and wholeness are here! I pray for the Holy Spirit to illuminate the minds of everyone reading these pages. I pray that each one may embrace this truth for themselves and their loved ones. We will look now at the specific roots of the autoimmune diseases that you or a loved one need to overcome!

Seven

THE SPIRITUAL ROOTS
OF HIGH BLOOD PRESSURE

Be careful [anxious] for nothing; but in every thing by
prayer and supplication with thanksgiving let your requests
be made known unto God. And the peace of God,
which passeth all understanding, shall keep your hearts
and minds through Christ Jesus.
—Philippians 4:6–7

There is excessive stress in America. That comes as no surprise! Twenty-five percent of adults in the United States have taken medication at some point for excessive stress and anxiety. Surveys have shown that 75 percent of employees believe that workers have more on-the-job stress than a generation ago. Workers report that job stress is more strongly associated with health complaints than any financial or family problems.[8]

8. "Workplace Stress," The American Institute of Stress, https://www.stress.org/workplace-stress.

In today's culture, in education, sports, business, even families with a domineering, controlling parent, everything is judged by performance. In our western society, we don't make provision for failure in the world, but God does. God says that a righteous man will fall and rise again: *"For a just man falleth seven times, and riseth up again: but the wicked shall fall into mischief"* (Proverbs 24:16). Again, *"Though he fall, he shall not be utterly cast down: for the Lord upholdeth him with his hand"* (Psalm 37:24). Paul reminds us in 2 Corinthians 12:10, *"For when I am weak, then am I strong."*

We don't make these allowances for failure in people because there's a stigma that everything must be a perfect performance. It's a pecking order, and only the elite survive in education and income while the rest of us are afraid we will fall by the wayside. That creates a lot of stress and anxiety in people. That stress is internalized and starts to affect our soul and our body systems.

OVERCOMING FEAR AND ANXIETY

Today, an estimated 103 million U.S. adults have high blood pressure. That's almost half of all adults in the United States![9] This is a plague that we can stop if we will embrace God's truth on how to overcome fear and anxiety in our lives. As we covered in chapter one, the spiritual roots of high blood pressure are fear, anxiety, and stress. At Be in Health, we understand that *stress*

---

9. Ted Handler, MD, "More than 103 Million Americans Will Have High Blood Pressure Under New Guidelines," *ABC News*, November 13, 2017, https://abcnews.go.com/Health/103-million-americans-high-blood-pressure-guidelines/story?id=51121618.

is just a *modern-day word for "fear."* The spirit of fear causes the cell walls of the arteries to stiffen and constrict, resulting in a narrowing of the blood vessels near the heart and a resistance to blood flow, increasing the pressure on the heart.

If you are diagnosed with high blood pressure, you will be prescribed pills that are called beta blockers. Although doctors know that hypertension is an anxiety/stress disorder, they don't tell you that. Instead, they'll give you a beta blocker. This medication will circumvent the imbalance of the sympathetic nervous system and get your cell membrane semi-rigidity to be broken and your blood pressure back to normal. The beta blockers cause the blood vessels to relax, which allows the blood to return to its natural flow. But does a beta blocker solve your spiritual problem? No, it doesn't, because you will still be bound by fear.

God's will is for you to get rid of fear, anxiety, and stress for good. That is why it is so important to understand how the spirit-soul-body connection, paired with temptation, affects your biology—why you must learn to cast down those temptations and unwanted thoughts of fear and stress from the enemy, repent to the Lord for embracing the law of sin, and renew your mind with the truths of God's Word by meditating on the Scriptures that tell us to "fear not" and "be anxious for nothing."

Now, I'm not telling you to stop taking your blood pressure medicine. But as you embrace the truth of God's Word and experience freedom from fear, your doctor may be eliminating that medicine from your life.

EXPOSING THE SPIRITUAL ROOTS

Over the years, I have discovered a very specific spiritual root associated with high blood pressure. It is the *fear of the future*, or the *fear of tomorrow*. In Luke 21:26, Jesus warns about the effects of fear: *"Men's hearts failing them for fear, and for looking after those things which are coming on the earth."* If you're taking thought for tomorrow, you are worrying! God provides the antidote in Matthew 6:34: *"Take therefore no thought for the morrow: for the morrow shall take thought for the things of itself. Sufficient unto the day is the evil thereof."*

When you begin to project into the future—about health, finances, or relationships—I call it being "scattered and smothered." Now, "scattered and smothered" might be something good at the Waffle House, but practicing it as a way of life will lead to significant consequences. If you are tormented by the fear of tomorrow, you are bound by anxious thoughts, speculating as to what might go wrong in the future to such an extent that you don't defeat anything today. This fear often projects the failures of your past into your future and robs you of the joy of today. But the Bible tells us, *"This is the day which the LORD hath made; we will rejoice and be glad in it"* (Psalm 118:24)!

If you're going to be victorious over this fear, apply your heart to righteousness today; tomorrow will take care of itself. *"Seek ye first the kingdom of God, and his righteousness; and all these things shall be added unto you"* (Matthew 6:33). That righteousness is His faith, not fear.

FEAR IS DEVIOUS

Fear is devious, and it can multiply; fear's main goal is to separate us from loving and trusting God. The spirit of fear can train us from our earliest existence to expect and dread rejection, to perform for approval, and to be afraid of what others may do to us or think about us. It trains us to develop mechanisms of self-protection in order to avoid the pain of these projected realities. With high blood pressure, in addition to the fear of the future, we have also seen the spiritual roots of fear of man, fear of failure, fear of rejection, and fear of poverty.

Fear of man will constantly have you looking to man rather than to God, seeking the approval of others. It's a form of idolatry because you place the opinion of others over the opinion of your heavenly Father. Fear of man can drive every decision, every action, and every motivation through a filter of what others will think or do. It often leads to withdrawal and isolation due to the dread of never measuring up to the expectations of those around you.

The Scriptures encourage us, *"The fear of man bringeth a snare: but whoso putteth his trust in the Lord shall be safe"* (Proverbs 29:25). God is the only person who will not fail us. He is steadfast and true. He is full of mercy, kindness, and compassion toward us. He is patient, and He is longsuffering with us. Above all, His love does not depend on our performance, does not falter in our failures, and remains strong on our behalf.

The fear of man often leads to *fear of failure*. Fear of failure provides no room for mistakes or humanness. It will paralyze you, inhibiting your ability to make choices or to engage in relationships. *Fear of rejection* causes you to continually speculate on who is going to reject you or how it will be done. If you fear rejection, you will be unable to develop your own identity. You will be too fearful to express your own opinions, beliefs, or values, and will be tempted to always just "follow the herd."

Fear of poverty, or fear of financial failure, is one of the greatest stressors in our society. The enemy will try to overwhelm you with fear of financial failure, along with the guilt and shame of financial mistakes. It ties in with the fear of the future, as it includes a projection of evil or bad things to come. Perhaps you continuously expect something to go wrong financially or that you will lose complete control of your finances. The root of the issue is that you may be deceived into listening to heavy, oppressive thoughts from the enemy concerning your financial situation. Perhaps you are trapped in a job you hate or in another financial situation where there appears to be no possible way to escape. The enemy wants you to feel hopeless and helpless so that you will give up rather than seek God for His ways. With God, there is always a way out. He is greater than any financial problems. And, as a good, loving Father, He wants to lead you to peace and joy in Him.

How should you deal with these fears of financial stress or ruin from the enemy? Deuteronomy 29:9 says, *"Keep therefore the words of this covenant, and do them, that ye may prosper in all that ye do."* Choose to submit your finances to God and trust Him with the outcome. Ask Him to forgive you for embracing the fear and shame of financial troubles. Even if you have made unwise financial decisions, His forgiveness is still available for you. When you release that heavy burden, your body can be at peace again, and that extra stress will stop interfering with your blood pressure! First Peter 5:7 says, "Casting all your care upon him; for he careth for you."

At Be in Health, we teach that the breakdown in relationship between God, ourselves, and others can lead to disease because the enemy—Satan—knows that if he can cause separation at any of these levels through fear, we are easy pickings. The spirit of fear will come disguised as a friend or a helper; it will offer us a false means of self-protection, security, and a sense of being in control. In reality, it is helping us build up walls around our heart to keep us in and others, even God, out. That's where the separation occurs. What is the result of these spirits of fear creating separation along with stress and anxiety in our lives? You may end up with a stress disorder—including high blood pressure.

What are stress disorders? They are illnesses or syndromes that are a result of fear, anxiety, stress, guilt, and shame. If you're struggling with any of these, you may have a disease or syndrome, or one may be on the way. In stress disorders, the enemy is out to control your nervous system. He will cause you to lose your peace by producing fearful thoughts affecting your central nervous system. You begin to feel pain, experience brain fog, and suffer a host of other symptoms, and then you need medication to manage it. High blood pressure is one of the most common stress disorders. (Fibromyalgia, chronic fatigue syndrome, diabetes 2, irritable bowel syndrome, and ulcerative colitis are other examples of stress disorders.)

STRESS: A MODERN-DAY WORD FOR "FEAR"

Have you ever been fearful? Have you seen a fearful person? They're dressed up in it. It's all over them. It has become an actual part of their personality. This is not from God. God has not given us a spirit of fear. The apostle Paul identified fear as a spirit: *"For God hath not given us **the spirit of fear**; but of power, and of love, and of a sound mind"* (2 Timothy 1:7).

There are many modern Bible translations that have changed the wording of this Scripture verse in 2 Timothy. They have replaced the phrase *"spirit of fear"* with the word *"timidity,"* leaving the *spirit* out altogether. This is denying the concept that fear is an *evil spirit* that wants to tempt you and control you. Fear is not just a psychological manifestation; it is an evil spirit that is plotting against us. God is the One who calls it the spirit of fear. We would be wise not to disagree with Him.

In the Old Testament, the book of Job also identifies fear as a spirit. *"Fear came upon me, and trembling, which made all my bones to shake. Then a spirit passed before my face; the hair of my flesh stood up: It stood still, but I could not discern the form thereof: an image was before mine eyes"* (Job 4:14–16). Fear is a spirit that comes from Satan's hidden kingdom.

According to Hebrew 11:1, *"**Faith** is the substance of things **hoped for**, the evidence of things not seen."* On the opposite side, *fear* is the substance of things we *do not* hope for! Fear is a powerful form of Satan's belief system. Faith is greater than fear. However, the two are equal in this one dimension: they both project into the future, and they both demand to be fulfilled.

Jesus said, "*According to your faith be it unto you*" (Matthew 9:29). The enemy wants to replace that with "According to your fear be it unto you."

Fear is an evil spirit that can influence your thoughts. Remember, 2 Timothy 1:7 says, "*For God hath not given us the **spirit** of fear; but of **power**, and of **love**, and of a **sound mind**.*" If you have unresolved fear, anxiety, and stress, you don't have any *power*. You don't have a *sound mind* because it is filled with stressful thoughts and imaginations. You're not able to give and receive *love* without fear. That's why 1 John 4:18 is such a powerful verse: "*There is no fear in love.*" If you don't feel love from childhood, you won't feel loved by other people as an adult. Guess what joins you in that vacuum of no love? The spirit of fear.

Fear works to prevent us from taking our struggles to our heavenly Father, who can help us properly process life's challenges. If we don't identify invasive thoughts as originating with the enemy and cast them down, we allow that spirit of fear to dwell in us and continually tempt us with fearful thoughts and feelings. "*Submit yourselves therefore to God. Resist the devil, and he will flee from you*" (James 4:7). That resistance often includes rebuking the spirit of fear, or the spirit of infirmity, in the name of Jesus.

Psalm 34:4 says, "*I sought the Lord, and he heard me, and **delivered me from all my fears**.*" If you seek the Lord and call upon His name, you will be delivered. That's a promise we should embrace. What happens if we embrace fear instead of faith in God and allow the spirit of fear to control our lives?

THE RESULTS OF FEAR ON YOUR IMMUNE SYSTEM

Your body is designed to serve you until something interferes with the design. Remember, when you don't cast down temptations from the spirit of fear, you internalize what you fear or dread, and you project that potential failure into the future. Your limbic system (involving the hippocampus, the amygdala, and the hypothalamus, as explained in chapter six) responds and senses that you're not at peace. As a result of fear, anxiety, stress, guilt, and shame, the hypothalamus causes misfired electrical and chemical signals to go out to the rest of the body and cause dis-ease of function in the endocrine system, the nervous system, and the digestive system—or in all these parts. One result is high blood pressure.

Most medical professionals agree that having a fearful outlook on life will negatively affect your health. Medical science recognizes that fear and emotional trauma change the brain, but, until recently, it was not certain that these were directly linked to causing primary hypertension. According to a September 2021 article published by the American Heart Association, recent studies report what we have been teaching for over twenty-five years: a constant stream of cortisol and other stress hormones will likely develop disease in stress-filled individuals—including high blood pressure. "Adults with normal blood pressure and high levels of stress hormones [including cortisol] were more likely to develop high blood pressure and experience cardiovascular events compared to those who had lower stress hormone levels."[10]

10. "Elevated Stress Hormones Linked to Higher Risk of High Blood Pressure and Heart Events," *Hypertension* Journal Report, Newsroom, September 13, 2021, https://newsroom.heart.org/news/elevated-stress-hormones-linked-to-higher-risk-of-high-blood-pressure-and-heart-events.

THE EFFECTS OF CORTISOL

Now we come to cortisol. I have been teaching for decades on the serious effects of cortisol on the immune system. Cortisol is a naturally occurring steroid released by the adrenal glands. As our primary stress hormone, it has an important function, especially to help us in "fight-or-flight" situations that could be dangerous. Now, the enemy wants us to believe that we are in danger continually, so he will feed us fearful thoughts that cause the unchecked release of cortisol into our body. What God created to help us fight an enemy has now turned on us and become a destroyer. It is the result of the spirit of fear attacking you with the end goal of weakening or destroying your immune system.

When you have unresolved fear, anxiety, and stress, cortisol is being released continuously. I like to call it a "cortisol drip" to help you understand how this cortisol release acts—like a leaky faucet. If you are unable to resolve the fear in your life, then the drip, drip of cortisol will begin to weaken your immune system. Cortisol does not compromise the immune system because of a lack of nutrition. Cortisol destroys the immune system because of fear. Now, this kind of fear is not generated by something like the fear of flying or the fear of spiders. It comes predominantly from major relationship breakdowns, such as the fear of failing others, the fear of rejection, and the fear of man, among other fears.

KEEP YOUR IMMUNE SYSTEM HEALTHY

How do you keep your immune system healthy? Recognize the spirits of fear and infirmity that you have allowed to take over your thought life. Repent to the Father for embracing the law of sin, and allow His love to affirm you. Allow God to develop His nature in you. The Holy Spirit is the third person of the Godhead and represents God's nature, among other things. For you to have an immune system like the one God created for you, your nature should express love, joy, peace, longsuffering, goodness, kindness, gentleness, faithfulness, and temperance! The Bible goes on to say there is no law that can defeat them. *"But the fruit of the Spirit is love, joy, peace, longsuffering, gentleness, goodness, faith, meekness, temperance: against such there is no law"* (Galatians 5:22–23). This nature of God in you is what produces a healthy immune system.

I want you to win this! For the sake of your health, get rid of as much fear as you can because God is not giving it to you; Satan is. Let the Holy Spirit form His incredible nature in you. The enemy might still tempt you, but he cannot touch you. Take ownership of your life! Renew your mind with His Word and rejoice in your freedom!

Eight

OVERCOMING FEAR, STRESS, AND ANXIETY

Men's hearts failing them for fear, and for looking after those things which are coming on the earth: for the powers of heaven shall be shaken.
—Luke 21:26

Many people think this Scripture only refers to something catastrophic happening in the future. But there is enough fear and anxiety in the world for this verse to apply to today, as well! Men and women's hearts are failing them because of fear. We are afraid of the future, afraid of one another, afraid of political outcomes, afraid of illness, and plagued with the fear of death. The first target organ for the spiritual roots of fear, anxiety, and stress is the heart and the arteries. Remember, the enemy cannot give you a cardiovascular disease through this fear and anxiety unless you give him permission. Jesus finished the work for us on the cross; now we need to follow it in obedience. It doesn't work out well for us when we try to follow Him in disobedience and want to be healed at the same time.

You are the one responsible for cause and effect. You are responsible to be a responder to God and His Word; you are not responsible to respond to the devil. Hebrews 5:14 says, *"Even those who by reason of use have their senses exercised to discern both good and evil."* Christians must learn to discern good from evil. You cannot say, "The devil made me do it." You have the responsibility to seek God's Word in order to make the right decision. That is cause and effect. The Bible says that *"in him we live, and move, and have our being"* (Acts 17:28). We live in this world, but we don't have to act like the world. Take on God's nature instead and repent from and put off Satan's nature that is creating disease in your body.

Here is the case study of a woman who was set free from the spiritual roots of fear and healed of high blood pressure.

"In the autumn of 2017, during my regular doctor's visits, my blood pressure readings were high. I didn't think much of it, but my doctor became concerned and asked me to monitor my blood pressure at home three times a day. When the readings remained higher than they should have been, the spirit of fear began to tempt me with anxious thoughts. I had been healed of another stress disorder, chronic fatigue syndrome, years earlier by walking out the biblical teachings that I received from Be in Health. I had been delivered from the spirits of fear, stress, and anxiety in my life. I was determined that I was not going to accept a new diagnosis. It was not going to become 'my high blood pressure.'

"One night, after an unfortunate evening spent with a very condemning Christian couple, I took my blood pressure, and it was *very* high. That, combined with the darkness and disappointment of the evening, sent me into a panic attack, which I had not had in a long while, nor since. My husband called 9-1-1, the ambulance arrived, and the medical attendants told me to take a Xanax and see my doctor. First, I called the Spiritual Lifeline at Be in Health and received ministry concerning God's desire to heal me; they also prayed against the schemes of the devil in my life.

"Six months later, my father almost died from a heart event. Heart disease and hypertension are generational in our family. The day I received the call about my father, my anxiety skyrocketed, and my blood pressure numbers rose accordingly. That week, my doctor diagnosed me with very high blood pressure and prescribed three different medications. I still wasn't going to give up on God's promise of healing, though; so, at that appointment, I made a confession of faith. I told the doctor that I would soon be off those medications because God had healed me before, and He would do it again! His response was kind, but he was certain that I would need the medication for the rest my life. My response startled him: 'No, I will not.'

"I called the Spiritual Lifeline at Be in Health once again so that they could stand with me in faith. While continuing to take my medication, I asked my heavenly Father for healing, claiming God's Word over my life. I prayed daily that the walls of my arteries would soften, and that my heart wouldn't need to work so hard to pump the blood through my veins.

"At each follow-up visit, I reminded the doctor and nurses that I would not be taking the medicine for long, that I was praying for the walls of my arteries to soften, and that I was standing on God's Word against fear and anxiety. I would get crazy looks from all of them!

"In August 2019, I had an unrelated surgery. When the physical therapist came to my home after the surgery, she took my blood pressure as part of her routine and told me that my pressure was low. A couple of weeks later, I began to feel extremely fatigued, more so than before the surgery. When I called the doctor, he told me to decrease the dosage of my medications and make an appointment soon.

"The fatigue continued, along with depression. I couldn't even walk to the mailbox. My husband and I prayed that God would reveal the cause of both. The following morning, my first thought was, 'Check your blood pressure.' That first reading was very low. When I called the doctor, gave him the blood pressure numbers, and described how badly I felt, he told me to stop the medications immediately and monitor my blood pressure throughout the day. During this same time, I realized that the fear and anxiety that had been tormenting me were gone and had been gone for weeks. Within days of stopping the medication, the fatigue lifted completely, and the depression was gone!

"Healing from disease does not always happen immediately, but when the Scripture proclaims that He is the God who forgives all our iniquities and heals all our diseases, we need to stand on that Word without wavering. (See Psalm 103:3.) Today, whenever the enemy tries to rear his head with fear in stressful situations, I remind myself of the truth of God's Word!"

—Julie P.

NO FEAR IN LOVE

The foundational Scripture we use for the healing of stress disorders is 1 John 4:18: *"There is no fear in love, but perfect love casteth out fear."* I can't emphasize enough that all spiritually rooted disease caused by any kind of fear involves a breach of relationship at some level. It could be a breach in your relationship with God; a breach in relationship with yourself, where you won't forgive yourself for your past; or a breach with someone else whom you can't forgive for hurting or abandoning you. *"He that sayeth he is in the light, and hateth his brother, is in darkness even until now"* (1 John 2:9).

Remember how you can recognize that you still are harboring unforgiveness or hatred toward someone else? If you feel a ping in your spirit every time you think of that person or persons, then you know something is wrong in your heart! Search your heart and allow the Holy Spirit to reveal any fear or breach in relationships for which you should repent. Cast down those temptations and thoughts that rise up against God's Word. Your Father loves you, and He has good things for your life—not rejection, fear, and disaster.

I'm aware of some people who have a huge breach in their relationships with others because of fear. Don't let this be you! Don't be ruled by the fear of man. *"The fear of man bringeth a* snare: but whoso putteth his trust in the LORD shall be safe" (Proverbs 29:25). Hebrews 13:6 tells us, *"The Lord is my helper, and I will not fear what man shall do unto me."* If you have this kind of fear of others, or of their opinion of you, you need to get it resolved. You need to have resolution, repentance, and restoration in your fellowship. Then, fear becomes a diminishing thought. It fades into the background because you're in fellowship. If fear is the underlying root of your stress syndrome, the syndrome will begin to fade away. Getting rid of fear in your life is a powerful gateway to your freedom from illness. You need to kick the spirit of fear to the curb, embrace the love of the Father, and let your immune system be restored to health!

Many people know that they have stress in their lives, but they don't know how to relieve it without medications. For every fear, there is a remedy found in the Word of God. When you lift a promise from the Scripture up over the temptation of the enemy, you will have blessings and victory. Two essential steps to overcome stress are *belief* and *perseverance*.

The number one thing is *to believe*. Will you choose to believe God and His Word today? The second most important thing is *to persevere*. It's not "one and done." It's a process to identify and work through each fear. As you continue to persevere, feelings of fear will become easier to identify. Through the process, you can have peace with yourself and your loving Father, knowing that He will be faithful to complete His good work in you. *"Being confident of this very thing, that he which hath begun a good work in you will perform it until the day of Jesus Christ"* (Philippians 1:6).

FREEDOM FROM DISEASE

The following testimony is of a husband and wife who are on the road to freedom from disease as they stand on God's Word.

"If you had told us about all of the change that would occur in our lives in just twelve months, we never would have believed you. There were so many areas of our lives that just felt 'stuck,' and we had accepted them as 'just the way things are.' Doug had hypertension, and his blood pressure was spiking to dangerous levels. He often felt hopeless and depressed, so fearful about the future. My chronic urinary tract infections had led to interstitial cystitis (an ongoing inflammatory condition in the bladder), and I was often in immense pain for days at a time. The only relief I had was from special medicine that had to be administered through a catheter. Both of us had incredible amounts of fear, anxiety, stress, and anger about all of the situations we found ourselves in. It was affecting our marriage and spilling over to our children.

"We had the book *A More Excellent Way* sitting on our bookshelf for thirteen years but never had any desire to look at it. Now, since we had already tried every other modality for healing, we figured it couldn't hurt. When we were finished reading, we knew we had to attend a For My Life retreat together. Even though we had been in Christian ministry for years, for the first time, we truly believed in the Father's love for us. We recognized many of the strongholds that were affecting us and our children, and we learned how to change through meaningful repentance combined with resisting Satan's law of sin.

"A lot happened in that first week, and we came home overflowing with hope. Back at home, we kept at it by putting the principles we had learned into practice. A couple of months later, I went back to Be in Health for the Walk Out Workshop and received great insight into how to overcome the strongholds of fear, rejection, and bitterness. We went back again for the family week, so that all four of our children could attend the kids' program and hear about the Father's love for themselves.

"Learning the truth about healing and disease through the Be in Health ministries completely changed our lives. Although we are still in the beginning of our journey, we are so grateful to have found these biblical truths in this season of our lives. Doug's blood pressure is much lower, he has been healed of food allergies, and he is more engaged in the godly order of our home. I am off all of my medication, and my bladder pain has subsided substantially. We know this journey of overcoming isn't always easy, but we are committed to knowing the Father's love and desire for us. And our lives are improving more and more every day."

—Doug and Carrie

SEVEN STEPS TO DEFEAT FEAR AND STRESS IN YOUR LIFE

1. **Stop:** When you feel symptoms associated with fear, stop and ask yourself, "What have I been listening to that is causing me to go into fight or flight?" *"For the word of God is quick, and powerful…and is a discerner of the thoughts and intents of the heart"* (Hebrews 4:12).

2. **Acknowledge:** This is not the time to go into denial. Maybe there really is a problem that needs to be dealt with. You can say something like this: "Yes, that may be a big problem, but I can't wait to see how God is going to handle it!" This attitude effectively puts your problem into God's hands with anticipation that He will work with you to help you fix it. You can be excited to see what He will do on your behalf! *"Casting all your care upon him; for he careth for you"* (1 Peter 5:7).

3. **Observe:** Write those suspicious thoughts down and take inventory of them. Ask God to show you the patterns that don't line up with His truth. *"…and bringing into captivity every thought to the obedience of Christ"* (2 Corinthians 10:5).

4. **Cast Down:** After you've recognized the enemy, renounce his ways of thinking, repent to God for believing them above His Word, and remove them. (See the "8 Rs to Freedom" in the "What's Next?" section of this book.) *"Casting down imaginations, and every high thing that exalteth itself against the knowledge of God…"* (2 Corinthians 10:5).

5. **Replace:** Ask God to help you find Scriptures that overturn the lies of the enemy in your life. *"And Jesus answered him, saying, It is written, That man shall not live by bread alone, but by every word of God"* (Luke 4:4).

6. **Believe:** Believe the Word of God and the leading of the Holy Spirit. *"Jesus said unto him, If thou canst believe, all things are possible to him that believeth"* (Mark 9:23).

7. **Repeat:** Persevere, don't give up, and don't let the enemy accuse you or condemn you if you fall down again. Proverbs 24:16 says, *"The just man falls seven times and rises up again."* So, keep on getting up, grab your Father's hand, and allow Him to help you recover yourself again.

Remember, the life of an overcomer is a journey, not a sprint. Learn how to enjoy the journey, and when something comes up, bring it to your Father with the expectation that He will help you defeat it. Look forward to the good fruit that will spring forth from your life as you continue to line your ways up with His. That fruit will be the blessings of righteousness: healing, peace, restoration in relationships, and provision for your life.

Nine

HEALING FOR THE HEART

Did you know that there are some heart malfunctions that are classified as heart disease but are not a disease at all? They are syndromes; the heart is malfunctioning although there is no organic problem behind it. In addition to hypertension, medical research shows that other cardiovascular diseases including angina, mitral valve prolapse, and arrhythmic heart problems are related to fear, anxiety, and stress. In the textbook *Pathophysiology: The Biologic Basis for Disease*, under the heading "Examples of Stress-Related Diseases and Conditions," diseases such as angina, arrhythmias, hypertension, and mitral valve prolapse are considered fear, anxiety, and stress disorders by the medical community.

Who said the same thing? God said it in Luke 21:26: *"Men's hearts failing them for fear, and for looking after those things which are coming on the earth."* Since God knows this, don't you think He wants us to know it, too? That is why the Bible directly links fear to heart problems. These insights into cardiovascular disease may be just what your heart needs to return to health and peace and to function the way God designed it to.

Unfortunately, it isn't just older adults who need to be aware of the effects of stress on blood pressure and the heart. Nearly two decades ago, the American Heart Association meeting report announced the following: "Young adults who fume at the slowpoke ahead of them on the freeway may be racing toward high blood pressure.... 'Time urgency/impatience (TUI) assessed during young adulthood is associated with increased risk of hypertension years later.'"[11]

HOW FEAR AND STRESS AFFECT YOUR HEART

We know that our body, including the heart, directly responds to our thoughts. *Angina pectoris* is a type of chest pain caused by reduced blood flow to the heart. It is severe pain in the chest associated with emotional stress and characterized by feelings of suffocation and apprehension. Patients feel a heaviness, pressure, or very painful spasms in the chest due to a thickening of the arteries near the heart. It is directly linked to the spiritual root of fear, anxiety, and stress which is causing constriction of the coronary arteries. When a person is struggling constantly with fearful and anxious thoughts, it can cause a constriction of the heart muscle. This makes it more difficult for the blood to travel freely through the blood vessels. This binding is what causes the pain of angina. The antidote is the Word of God. "*The Lord is my rock, and my fortress, and my deliverer; my God, my strength, in whom I will trust; my buckler, and the horn of my salvation, and my high tower*" (Psalm 18:2).

11. American Heart Association, "Want Hypertension? Hurry Up!" EurekAlert!, November 20, 2002, https://www.eurekalert.org/news-releases/515725.

Mitral valve prolapse can be caused by congenital defects or infections. But in many cases, we have found that the mitral valve doesn't close smoothly due to neurological misfirings. The misfiring interrupts the electrical connection to the valve. It is the reality of fear, anxiety, and stress in the spirit and the soul that launches the sequence of events that causes an interruption of the electrical connection to the valve. Once again, the possible spiritual roots for the misfiring are fear, anxiety, and stress.

Heart arrhythmias are due to an electrical breakdown in the heart rate. They are often disturbances of the heart rhythm caused by the spiritual roots of fear, anxiety, and stress. Not only can the heart be stimulated by chemical messengers, through the involuntary nervous system; it is also neurologically sensitive to thought via what the medical community refers to as the mind-body connection. We understand that it is actually a *spirit-soul-body* connection. And the disturbances that wrong thoughts can cause to your body systems is the reason that the cardiovascular system does not receive the correct electrical signals and the heartbeat is interrupted. The heart organ itself is not damaged, but there has been a disruption in its proper function. We have observed many people healed of heart arrythmia when they have overcome the fear, anxiety, and stress in their lives. Amy is one of those case histories.

A HEALED HEART

This is the recent testimony of a woman healed of heart arrythmia.

"When I was diagnosed with heart arrythmia, I was afraid. I called a friend who I knew had faith in God for healing. Immediately, she recommended Dr. Wright's book *A More Excellent Way*. I read the book and was amazed at how quickly I recognized the spirit of fear that had been overwhelming my own life. When I repented and turned toward God for forgiveness and peace, I was healed from the heart arrythmias—and it has never returned!

"I read *A More Excellent Way* a few more times so that I would get the biblical encouragement I needed to continue in my freedom from fear. In 2017, I learned about the For My Life retreat in Thomaston, Georgia, so I traveled there from Texas. During the week at the retreat, I was immersed in the truth of God's Word and the power of standing against the enemy's lies, and I received great freedom from fear. For the first time, I heard of the powerful effects that bitterness and unforgiveness can have against our bodies. I let go of some bitterness that I never realized was there. I felt so much better, and I was excited to share these truths with my children and even my grandchildren.

"Jesus gave His life to save us for eternity; He also suffered to bring healing to our bodies on earth. When you see healing in your own life, you are so grateful, and you want to share it with other people. The biggest thing I learned through my time at Be in Health was that God created our bodies to heal themselves. We are an incredible creation. If you stop beating yourself up with fear, anxiety, and stress, and you forgive others, your body will begin the healing process. The healing begins when you get rid of the junk! You are worth the time to get to know the truth of God's promises and what Jesus has accomplished on your behalf!"

—Amy K.

DOWN THE FAMILY TREE

The medical community recognizes that many of these heart diseases follow family trees through the generations. They often see the same condition affecting a person that affected their parents and even their grandparents before them. There is evidence in some of these situations of genetic markers leading to a predisposition to these diseases. But I want to submit that a genetic predisposition can actually be a spiritual predisposition, as well!

From my observation, a spirit of fear, anxiety, and stress can track with the generations just as any other type of iniquity can. It becomes a learned behavior that is so familiar that many of us don't even know or recognize the difference. It looks like this: perhaps a grandparent struggled with fear, stress, and anxiety, then their children learned and came into agreement with that same pattern of thinking and then, in turn, passed it on to their children. We are reminded in Numbers 14:18 that *"the Lord is longsuffering, and of great mercy, forgiving iniquity and transgression, and by no means clearing the guilty, visiting the iniquity of the fathers upon the children unto the third and fourth generation."*

A spirit of fear will take whatever open door it can *into the next generation* in order to program and train each person in its ways. It can even come in from the womb if the mother is struggling with fear and stress during her pregnancy. God holds the keys to releasing you and your subsequent generations from the consequences of iniquity. If you ask Him and seek Him about it, He truly will deliver you from all your fears.

GOD WANTS TO LEAD US

We have discussed the types of heart disease that are directly linked to a spirit of fear. The next question is this: How do we deal with this fear issue so that our hearts can return to health? God doesn't just want to root up the iniquity in our lives; He wants to lead us in His ways and form us in His image so that we can walk in health and in the fruit of His Spirit. We are so thankful that, at Be in Health, by God's grace, we have been given answers to the healing of disease from the inside out.

Below are two testimonies of the healing power we can receive from God when we recognize the roots of fear, stress, and anxiety in our lives, and turn to the Father for His forgiveness and restoration.

"Last year, one of my coworkers was testing his blood pressure at work, and he jokingly asked if I wanted to test mine, too. I decided to do it and was shocked that my blood pressure numbers were alarmingly high. My coworker recommended that I see a doctor to find out what was going on. I've always been very healthy and had never had any serious health issues, so this was very difficult for me. The doctor diagnosed me with hypertension and prescribed blood pressure medication.

"My wife and I were familiar with the teachings at Be in Health, so we began praying that God would show me the spiritual roots of the issue, asking Him to give me the wisdom I needed to overcome high blood pressure. In the meantime, I began regulating my diet, reducing my salt intake, and eating smaller portions. I knew the Scriptures said that our bodies are the temple of the Holy Spirit, so I wanted to honor the Lord. The diet changes helped some, but my blood pressure was still high.

"A few months later, I attended a For My Life retreat, and one of the teachers shared their own journey of overcoming hypertension. He had worked in a similar industry, so I really related to his story. During that week, God revealed several issues in my life. I was trying to hold everything together at work and at home, believing the enemy's lie that if I didn't do everything myself, no one would get it done. God convicted me that it wasn't my responsibility to try to hold everything together—it was His. After the retreat, it was a process of learning to trust God with my life and not take on the burden of responsibility for everything. I was even able to release some responsibilities to others.

"This revelation also helped me overcome the perfectionism I had taken on in our marriage. So often, I projected my fears of not being perfect onto my wife, which made her feel like she couldn't do anything well enough to please me. That wasn't my heart, but that's what my perfectionism had done to her. God also revealed that I harbored a fear of man and the opinion of others. As I've been able to let go of these things, confessing them as sin to the Father and not allowing my identity to get wrapped up in what I accomplish, it has brought a new freedom into my life. I have been released from a tremendous burden that I wasn't even aware I was carrying.

"Since then, I have been slowly weaned off the high blood pressure medication. Eventually, my numbers were so good that I no longer needed the medication at all. I still test my blood pressure regularly. Now that I am aware of the effects the enemy can have on my health, I guard against the thoughts and circumstances he uses to try to bring fear and anxiety back into my life. At those times, I pay close attention to the thoughts I've been listening to, cast them down, surrender my life to God, and recover myself again.

"My wife and I are so grateful for God's faithfulness to give me the revelation and understanding I needed to be healed of high blood pressure. It's taken a tremendous burden off both of us and brought new freedom into our lives!"

—John M.

"Hypertension is a disease that often has no symptoms; I had no idea that I had it. Eleven years ago, the high blood pressure, along with some family history of hypertension, led to my having a stroke. As I was recovering, my husband and I took a close look at both the physical and spiritual realities of what was going on in my life. We had been embracing the biblical teachings of Be in Health in our church for years, and now we would be putting them into practice very personally.

"After the stroke, the first thing my husband and I did was address the possible spiritual roots. We prayed for the Lord to reveal the spiritual cause of fear and anxiety in my life. Sometimes, when there is fear in your life, it leads to overeating. Even overeating can have a spiritual root. When we are anxiety-ridden, we often turn to food for comfort rather than turning to God, whom the Bible calls 'the God of all comfort': 'Blessed be God, even the Father of our Lord Jesus Christ, the Father of mercies, and the God of all comfort' (2 Corinthians 1:3). When I was anxious or fearful, I would turn to food for temporary relief, when I should have been turning to the Lord for my comfort and strength. Being overweight is another factor that can lead to a diagnosis of high blood pressure. I needed to treat my body as the temple of the Holy Spirit and control my overeating.

"On this journey, we discovered that the spirit of perfectionism—trying to be perfect—was the primary root behind my stress, but I didn't recognize it right away. Perfectionism is when you believe that you are the only one who can do anything correctly in your circle of activities. My inner thought was, 'If I don't do it, it won't be done right.' If someone did something I didn't like, including my husband, I would have to redo it. Perfectionism comes from the enemy because no one can be perfect. In your thoughts, the enemy gives you a goal that you can't possibly reach for the express purpose of bringing fear and anxiety into your life. Perfectionism and fear work together.

"Right after the stroke, my husband had to do everything for me. I should have been grateful for his help, but his efforts still weren't good enough for me, and I complained that he wasn't doing things correctly. I just didn't understand the spirit of perfectionism that was driving me.

"Then, our daughter came for a visit. When she saw what was going on, she said, 'Mom, what is wrong with you? You have a husband to serve you in love at this deep level, and you're complaining to him that he's not doing it right! You've got to get a grip, Mom!' That is when I realized that it was the spirit of perfectionism that was driving my stress and anxiety.

"How did I overcome high blood pressure? I addressed the spiritual issue of perfectionism, confessing it as sin, and I began to trust in God. My husband and I both lost weight. Slowly, my medication was decreased. First, it was cut in half, and we closely monitored my blood pressure. Then, it was cut in half again. Each time, my blood pressure numbers remained healthy. Finally, I was able to get off the medication completely. That was over a decade ago. For the last ten and a half years, I have been off blood pressure medication, walking in my healing, and rejoicing in my freedom in God!"

—Jodie P.

A MORE EXCELLENT WAY

How do we get healed of this "incurable" disease of high blood pressure? By recognizing the fear in our lives, taking responsibility, and repenting to God for allowing it to control us. That's good theology. The other road is cohabiting with fear and all the disease management that rides along with it. When you are able to call the fear of tomorrow a sin, and then take your peace from God's Word, guess what your blood vessels will do? They will relax! Blood will be able to flow properly again, and the curse of high blood pressure will be vanquished forever. The fruit of your life is dependent upon whether you yield to faith or fear. Faith brings life to the heart, while fear may bring the heart some serious short-circuiting!

The Word of God is your sword of the Spirit to fight the enemy, to fight the law of sin that attempts to take over your life. (See Ephesians 6:10–18.) Here are just a few Scripture verses to renew your mind and release you from the bondage of the enemy's fear-filled lies. Let the Holy Spirit bring freedom to you through God's Word.

What time I am afraid, I will trust in thee.   (Psalm 56:3)

Fear not: for I have redeemed thee, I have called thee by thy name; thou art mine.   (Isaiah 43:1)

The LORD is my light and my salvation; whom shall I fear? the LORD is the strength of my life; of whom shall I be afraid?   (Psalm 27:1)

The LORD is on my side; I will not fear: what can man do unto me?   (Psalm 118:6)

And he laid his right hand upon me, saying unto me, Fear not; I am the first and the last.   (Revelation 1:17)

Peace I leave with you, my peace I give unto you: not as the world giveth, give I unto you. Let not your heart be troubled, neither let it be afraid.   (John 14:27)

WHAT'S NEXT?

Bless the Lord, O my soul, and forget not all his benefits:
who forgiveth all thine iniquities;
who healeth all thy diseases.
—Psalm 103:2–3

We have taken a journey together to expose the spiritual roots of diseases through the knowledge of biblical truth. Let's review a few of these foundational truths concerning the healing of disease.

First, spiritually rooted disease is a result of separation from God, separation from yourself, or separation from others. Therefore, all healing of spiritually rooted diseases begins with reconciliation with God—receiving His love, embracing Him as your Father, and making your peace with Him. Reconciliation with yourself and with others are the next essential steps.

Second, we recognize that there are two kingdoms waging war on the inside of us: the law of sin and the law of God. Remember, the apostle Paul expressed our need to be set free from the temptations and the root of sin in our lives through Jesus Christ: *"O wretched man that I am! who shall deliver me from the body of this death? I thank God through Jesus Christ our Lord"* (Romans 7:24–25).

Third, once we are delivered from these roots, it becomes our responsibility to renew our minds and change those old patterns of ungodly thinking. Casting down evil imaginations and filling yourself with the Word of God in your thought life is your responsibility. *"Casting down imaginations, and every high thing that exalteth itself against the knowledge of God, and bringing into captivity every thought to the obedience of Christ"* (2 Corinthians 10:5).

At Be in Health, we call this process Walk Out. We even have a retreat called Walk Out Workshop, or WOW, because we know how important it is to walk out the process of our sanctification and stay on track with the biblical truths that set us free from disease.

THE 8 RS TO FREEDOM

We also teach what we call the "8 Rs to Freedom."[12] It's vital for you to remember and apply these principles. Post them where you can see them daily, such as on your refrigerator or your

---

12. See Henry W. Wright, *A More Excellent Way* (New Kensington, PA: Whitaker House, 2009), 161–169.

bathroom mirror. Mostly important, post them on your heart. They are the pathway to your freedom!

1. **Recognize.** *You must recognize what it is.* Recognize the root problem(s) in your life: bitterness, hatred, fear, anxiety, anger, hostility, self-hatred, etc. Pray for discernment from the Holy Spirit. Discern good from evil in your life.

2. **Responsibility.** *You must take responsibility for what you recognize.* Not everybody wants to take responsibility after they recognize the problem. You need to take responsibility. God will walk alongside you, but He won't do it for you!

3. **Repent.** *Repent to God for participating in what you recognize.* The Bible tells us, *"Repent ye therefore, and be converted, that your sins may be blotted out, when the times of refreshing shall come from the presence of the Lord"* (Acts 3:19). Some people get mad at me when I tell them they need to repent to be free from disease. If you go to a doctor to find out why you are sick and how to get better, would you be offended if he told you the truth? Then, please, do not be offended if I tell you the truth. I love you, and I care what happens to you. I'm teaching you how to defeat evil spirits and disease.

4. **Renounce.** *You must make what you recognize your enemy and renounce it.* To repent literally means "to turn away from." Consider your past root of sin as your enemy, and renounce it! Some people have remorse, but they do not change on the inside. They

don't turn away from their sin. But I want you to get away from evil—as fast as you can. Love yourself, but hate the evil!

5. **Remove it.** *Get rid of it, once and for all!* Say to the law of sin within you, "Not only do I renounce you, but you and I cannot exist at the same place and the same time together." *"Cast away from you all your transgressions, whereby ye have transgressed; and make you a new heart and a new spirit"* (Ezekiel 18:31). Get that law of sin out of your face, and let God give you a new heart and spirit.

6. **Resist.** *When it tries to come back, resist it!* James 4:7 tells us that we are to submit ourselves to God and resist the devil: *"Submit yourselves therefore to God. Resist the devil, and he will flee from you."* Which one comes first? Submitting to God. Only then will you have the power to resist the enemy, not before. Whatever you have dealt with will try to come back. That is why we need God and each other to resist it.

7. **Rejoice.** *Give God thanks for setting you free.* Give God glory for your freedom! Praise Him that you have experienced grace and mercy from a living God who loves you. He is worthy of your praise!

8. **Restore.** *Help someone else get free.* After you have received the blessings of God, it's time for you to begin helping to restore others. Part of restoring is bringing the gospel to those you love, instructing those who are separated from the refreshing of the Lord, and

discipling them in freedom from disease. *"That there should be no schism in the body; but that the members should have the same care for one another. And whether one member suffer, all the members suffer with it; or one member be honoured, all the members rejoice with it"* (1 Corinthians 12:25–26).

CHANGED INTO GOD'S IMAGE

Never forget that you are being changed into God's image as you follow His Word. *"But we all, with open face beholding as in a glass the glory of the Lord, are changed into the same image from glory to glory, even as by the Spirit of the Lord"* (2 Corinthians 3:18). Don't let anyone steal the truths that you have learned here. People with unbelief will try to debate you, discourage you, and drag you down to their image. You are not being formed into the image of any other person! You're being transformed into the image of God! As you are being changed into His image, you can expect Him to heal you of the diseases of the enemy because God honors His Word and His image. He honors who He is in you, not at the head level but at the heart level.

Through Jesus Christ, the Father is recapturing and recovering what He lost in the tragedy of the garden of Eden—His image in mankind. You are a product of that recovery and restoration. You are being called out of darkness and being changed into His marvelous light. *"But ye are a chosen generation, a royal priesthood, an holy nation, a peculiar people; that ye should shew forth the praises of him who hath called you out of darkness into his marvellous light*" (1 Peter 2:9). But you cannot be transformed unless you are reformed by the Word, because "*faith cometh by an holy hearing, and hearing by the Word of God*" (Romans 10:17).

FOLLOW THROUGH TO DEFEAT THE ENEMY!

I want to encourage you to follow through with your complete freedom from disease. Don't let the enemy discourage you. Everybody wants to be prayed for, but not everyone will follow up by defeating the lies of the enemy and embracing God's truth. Remember this Scripture: "*Ye shall know the truth, and the truth shall make you free*" (John 8:32). What I have been teaching you is designed to give you the truth and the faith to believe. This is not blind faith but real faith based on the knowledge of a living God revealed in the Bible. Your freedom was paid for over two thousand years ago on the cross, and the power of God was released into your life so that you could live in freedom. The Creator of the universe—your heavenly Father—wants you to be free!

> *Before I formed thee in the belly I knew thee; and before thou camest forth out of the womb I sanctified thee.*
>
> (Jeremiah 1:5)

> *But now thus saith the LORD that created thee, O Jacob, and he that formed thee, O Israel, Fear not: for I have redeemed thee, I have called thee by thy name; thou art mine.*
>
> (Isaiah 43:1)

Receive this prayer:

Father, I come to You in the name of Jesus. I want to thank You for those who have taken the time to read this book. I know from Psalm 139 in Your Word that they are fearfully and wonderfully made, and Your hand is upon each and every one of them. I know that I have given them many things to think about from Your Word. I ask You to release Your Holy Spirit to bring understanding and conviction, so that they may be changed from the inside out, and that diseases would vanish.

Father, we are just people, men and women from many different backgrounds. We have listened to lies we didn't know were lies; we have pursued courses we thought were right but are leading to our destruction. Please show us the good way where there is rest for our souls. Teach us to grow up in this thing called life and mature as sons and daughters of God. Let this be, Father, so that we may be whole in spirit, soul, and body, and that the generations after us would also be whole and a light to the world of Your glory and goodness and love toward us. Thank You so much for Your mercy, Sir, and continue to teach us by Your grace. In Jesus's name I pray. Amen.

WHAT BE IN HEALTH OFFERS

Now that we've exposed the spiritual roots of high blood pressure, you may be interested in these other resources that Be in Health® has to offer:

FOR MY LIFE®

For My Life is a one-week retreat hosted by Be in Health at our campus in Thomaston, Georgia. It is designed to help people who are seeking healing and restoration of their physical, emotional, and spiritual health. We believe that most diseases result from separation in relationship from God, ourselves, and others. This retreat will help you to identify and deal with the root issues that may be keeping you from being in health.

The For My Life retreat consists of intensive teachings, group ministry sessions, time to interact with the teachers and ask questions, and a time for personal prayer for healing at the end of the week. Be in Health endeavors to make For My Life a safe place for you to find hope and healing for your life.

WALK OUT® WORKSHOP (WOW)

After For My Life, the next step is the Walk Out Workshop (WOW). The term "walk out" refers to the journey of walking out of the old life of disease and hopelessness and entering into a new life of health and wholeness. During this one-week workshop, our team and attendees roll up their sleeves and begin to get really interactive with the principles from For My Life.

We address topics such as how to not go into guilt when we fall short, becoming established in our identity, overcoming temptation, how to forgive when you've been hurt, and learning to walk in the Father's love. Break-out groups, lots of Q & A, and continued healing of your spirit, soul, and body are all part of this amazing week.

FOR MY LIFE® EXPANDED (4MLX)

The For My Life eXpanded Retreat is our brand-new, next in series, five-day retreat, which will take you even deeper into the Be in Health teachings. Develop a profound understanding of the specific spiritual roots of major disease classes and discover powerful insights into healing and recovery in God. This retreat will set you on the next level of your overcomer journey. There are also corporate times of ministry throughout the week.

FOR MY LIFE® KIDS AND FOR MY LIFE® YOUTH

Every year in June and July, we offer For My Life for the whole family; that is the For My Life Adult, For My Life Youth (ages 13–17), and For My Life Kids (ages 6–12) Retreats all in the same week! This is an opportunity for the whole family to be transformed and healed from the inside out.

We hear so many people say, "If only I had known this when I was younger, I would have been saved from so much torment and heartache!" We've listened and developed these specialized retreats to continue our mission of establishing generations of overcomers. In the For My Life family week, everybody in the family can benefit and be on the same page spiritually. We take the same information that is presented in the adult For My Life Retreat but reformat it to be relevant and engaging for each audience.

WOW KIDS

After the For My Life family weeks, we have the WOW family weeks. This is an opportunity for the whole family to come and learn how to be overcomers together. The WOW Kids class (ages 6–12) will equip your children with the skills that they need to be overcomers. With a fun, engaging format, games, activities, and special "tools for freedom," your kids are sure to have a blast, make lasting memories, make new friends, and come out with valuable resources that will help them on their overcomer journey throughout their lives.

 To learn more about the Be in Health Retreats, visit: www.beinhealth.com/for-my-life

THE OVERCOMERS' COMMUNITY®

The journey of being an overcomer can be challenging, and we don't want you to have to do it alone. That is why we've developed the Overcomers' Community. This is a membership-based online forum dedicated to being a safe place for you to connect with the Be in Health Team as well as with other overcomers. You can ask questions, get support and encouragement, share testimonies, find specific spiritual roots of diseases, have access to a wide selection of complete teachings, access our private Facebook page, and more! We look forward to joining you and assisting you in your walk-out journey. With God's help, we can do this together!

 To learn more about the Overcomers' Community, visit: www.beinhealth.com/ overcomers-community

BE IN HEALTH® CONFERENCES NEAR YOU

Our Be in Health Team travels too! We bring one- to three-day conferences to locations all over the world. If you want to find out more about these conferences and when one might be held in your area, or if you are interested in helping us bring a conference to your area, go to: www.beinhealth.com

SPIRITUAL LIFELINE®

Spiritual Lifeline is a ministry of love and personal assistance from the Be in Health team; it is our most individualized form of ministry to you. Our Father promises to deliver us from the enemy as we apply His Word. Together, we'll look at God's plan for your situation and His promises that will sustain you. Private ministry and prayer sessions are provided over the phone or through an online voice- or video-calling platform.

Spiritual Lifeline is not a starting place at Be in Health. It is designed to come alongside and assist those who have previously attended our For My Life Retreat or have read and are applying the principles of Dr. Wright's books *A More Excellent Way* and *Exposing the Spiritual Roots of Disease*.

 To learn more about Spiritual Lifeline visit: www. beinhealth.com/phone-ministry

HEALTH RESOURCES

You can find all the information that we offer on specific disease and mental health topics. Under each topic, all the relevant Be in Health teachings, conferences, blogs, YouTube videos, healing testimonies, and related resources are categorized so you can find everything you need in one place. We continue to add new content, so keep checking back for more of the information you are looking for!

 Discover our Health Resources at: www.beinhealth. com/healing-resources

BE IN HEALTH® BOOKSTORE

If you enjoyed this book, you will love our other books and teaching resources in the Be in Health Bookstore. You will find an extensive selection of materials by Dr. Henry W. Wright, Pastor Donna Wright, and other leadership team members.

Topics range from the possible spiritual roots of diseases to how to overcome specific spiritual issues to teachings on sound biblical doctrine.

Dr. Henry W. Wright's book *A More Excellent Way* is our number one resource, selling over 300,000 copies worldwide. It is an excellent, comprehensive introduction to the root causes behind diseases and how to overcome them in your life. Included in the back of the book are 150 healing testimonies and a free teaching DVD.

In *Exposing the Spiritual Roots of Disease*, Dr. Wright presents a thoroughly biblical and compelling case for healing. If you think you've read all you need to know about healing, it's time to take another look! Dr. Wright clearly shows that disease is not a random occurrence and that science and medicine have their place in dealing with illness but can only offer disease management. What if the answers to true healing have been in the Bible all along?

Find these books and more in the Be in Health Bookstore: resources.beinhealth.com

BE IN HEALTH® BLOG

The Be in Health Blog offers biblical insights in a selection of articles about spiritual principles, overcoming, roots to diseases, and more. In addition, there are inspiring testimonies that are sure to encourage you in your own overcoming journey.

Find our blog at: www.beinhealth.com/blog

HOPE OF THE GENERATIONS CHURCH

Be in Health is a ministry of Hope of the Generations Church (HOGC), a local body of believers located in Thomaston, Georgia. HOGC is a nondenominational church and follows the model of the first-century church that was set in place by the apostles. We believe that every church, regardless of its background or diversity, should witness the same things recorded in the Bible: signs, wonders, healings, and miracles. These are life-altering tools of God to establish the authenticity of His Word.

Join us Sunday mornings at 10:00 a.m. EST or Friday nights at 7:00 p.m. EST.

 We also stream our church services on our YouTube channel: www.youtube.com/beinhealth

A.C.T.S. GLOBAL:
ASSOCIATION OF CHURCHES TEACHING AND SERVING®

Have you considered that God may be calling you to start, pastor, and establish a local church or gathering? Have the teachings of Be in Health opened your eyes, and now you want to tell others? Do you love people and want to see God's best for their lives?

Do you have a desire to guard the purity of the Bible and share that with others? Do you already, or do you desire to, gather people together to grow, heal, and fellowship together?

Do people come to you for help and direction for their lives? Are you ready to be a pastor but are held back by a lack of resources and training?

If you answered yes to one or more of these questions, A.C.T.S. Global is here to help you take the next step.

 To learn more about A.C.T.S. Global visit: www.actsglobal.com

BE IN HEALTH® E-MAIL LIST

Do you want to stay connected with Be in Health and receive updates, messages from our pastors, news, events, and blog posts directly in your inbox?

 Sign up for Be in Health's mailing list at: www.beinhealth.com

SOCIAL MEDIA

You can also follow us on your favorite social media platform!

Facebook: @beinhealth

Instagram: beinhealth

Twitter: @BeinHealth

YouTube: www.youtube.com/beinhealth

Pinterest: bnhealth

ABOUT THE AUTHOR

Dr. Henry W. Wright (1944–2019) was the senior pastor of Hope of the Generations Church in Thomaston, Georgia, and the president and founder of Be in Health® Global. Be in Health is a ministry that teaches on the spiritual roots of disease and blocks to healing, and hosts the world-renowned For My Life® Retreat.

Wright presented conferences worldwide and across broad denominational lines for over twenty-five years. Recognized for his understanding of disease from a spiritual perspective, he was a frequent guest on many well-known television and radio programs.

Wright was exposed to the power of God's healing at an early age when his mother was miraculously cured of terminal cancer and a fatal tumor that was wrapped around her jugular vein. Paralyzed and dying, she was carried to a church service where she cried out to God for healing so that she could raise her son. She repented of bitterness and made a Hannah-type covenant that she would raise him in the knowledge of God if

He would heal her. God healed her instantly and completely, breaking a genetic pattern of cancer that had been present in her family for generations.

Wright was committed to the belief that human problems are fundamentally spiritual, with associated physical and psychological manifestations. With his insights into the medical as well as the spiritual aspects of disease, he brought a fresh perspective to the process of ministering to the sick. He applied these principles successfully in bringing God's healing to people with a broad range of diseases, many of which were considered incurable.

Under the leadership of his wife, Pastor Donna Wright, and the elders of Hope of the Generations Church, Be in Health continues to carry on Dr. Wright's vision and ministry.